Love Without Becoming the Therapist

How to Support a Traumatized Partner, Protect Your Wellbeing, and Keep Love Mutual

Calvin Larkin Tanner

This book is for general information and education. It is not therapy, medical advice, or a substitute for care from a qualified professional. Reading it does not create a therapeutic or professional relationship between you and the author. If you or your partner are dealing with post-traumatic stress, complex trauma, depression, substance use, or any other health concern, please consult a licensed clinician who can assess your situation directly. Nothing here is intended to diagnose any person or to promise any particular result.

The stories in this book are fictional composites. Names are drawn from an invented name bank and belong to no real person. Any resemblance to a specific individual is coincidental. Details have been combined and altered so that the examples teach a point without exposing anyone's private life.

Some sections describe threats, coercion, and violence. If your safety or your partner's safety is at risk, contact local emergency services or a domestic violence hotline. In the United States, the National Domestic Violence Hotline can be reached at 800-799-7233. Support lines and their availability change over time, so confirm current local resources for your area.

The author and any affiliated parties disclaim liability for loss or risk, personal or otherwise, incurred as a consequence of the use or application of any content in this book. Wording that touches on legal or safety matters may vary by jurisdiction and should be reviewed with a qualified professional where it matters to your circumstances.

First Edition, 2026.

ISBN; 979-8-90678-172-7

Staten House

Table of Contents

About the Author

Calvin Larkin Tanner is a researcher who studies how trauma shapes close relationships. He writes practical, warm guides for the people standing beside someone in recovery, in the belief that partners deserve real instruction and not just encouragement. Love Without Becoming the Therapist grew out of that conviction. The chapters that follow are an attempt to give those partners a clearer map and a lighter load.

Preface

Research on post-traumatic stress has widened well beyond the person who carries the diagnosis. Studies of couples now show that trauma reaches the partner too, shaping how they behave, what they take on, and how much of the relationship reorganizes itself around symptoms. Clinicians even have a term for the way a caring partner adjusts their own conduct to lower a loved one's distress: partner accommodation. What the public conversation still lacks is a practical account of how to support a traumatized partner before that accommodation quietly consumes the supporter.

This book offers one. Its central model sorts the work of a strained relationship into three columns: what belongs to you, what belongs to your partner, and what the two of you hold together. That sorting matters, because the most common difficulty supporting partners face is not a shortage of love but a steady drift across those lines, taking on responsibilities that were never theirs to hold. The approach is not codependency recovery, and it does not cast the supporter as the problem. It addresses a specific, correctable pattern of over-functioning.

That pattern has a recognizable shape. A partner begins managing moods, watching for triggers, screening plans, and running an informal treatment program at home, and over months the relationship narrows into a clinic. Most people in this position cannot say where support ends and management begins, cannot find guidance that treats them as a partner rather than as a caregiver in a manual, and are left to improvise a role no one prepared them for.

This book sets out to correct that. Applying the three-column model across ten chapters, it shows how to help without taking over, how to set boundaries that protect a relationship rather than punish it, how to talk about professional treatment without becoming the treatment, and how to keep care moving in both directions. The aim is practical. A reader should finish able to support a partner as a partner, with their own wellbeing intact.

It is written to stand on its own, though it sits comfortably beside other practical guides for people supporting a loved one through a hard season, and it holds its focus tightly on the supporting partner's position rather than on clinical treatment itself. Its primary readers are the partners of people living with PTSD or complex trauma, especially those who have slid into the role of rescuer or unpaid therapist. Therapists, counselors, and group facilitators who work with such couples will also find a framework they can put directly into a client's hands.

What follows is not therapy, not a diagnosis, and not a guarantee that a relationship can be saved or a partner healed. Some situations, including those marked by coercion or violence, call for specialized help that no book can replace, and the final chapter says so without hedging. Within those limits, the intent here is plain: to help a caring partner support someone they love without disappearing inside the effort.

Introduction

You did not decide to become your partner's therapist. That is the strange part. There was no evening when you sat down and agreed to monitor their mood from across a room, to plan the week around what might set them off, to answer the three in the morning panic, to call in sick on their behalf, to become the person who holds everything together while looking, to the outside world, completely fine. It happened by degrees. Love asked for a small thing, and then a slightly larger thing, and you said yes each time because saying yes is what love does. Somewhere in that chain of small yeses, the shape of the relationship changed, and one day you noticed that you were no longer only a partner. You had also become a manager, a mediator, an appointment reminder, a crisis line, and a shock absorber, and you were tired in a way that sleep did not fix.

If any of that lands, this book is for you. It is for the person who loves someone with post-traumatic stress or complex trauma and who has slowly taken on a role that does not belong to any partner: the role of unpaid clinician. You may be thirty or fifty-five. You may be a wife, a husband, a partner of any gender. Your person may be a veteran, a survivor of assault or abuse, someone who lived through an accident or a loss or a childhood that no child should have. The specifics differ. The private question tends to be the same. How can I be loving without disappearing into my partner's trauma?

Here is the promise of this book, stated plainly and without exaggeration. You can support your partner as a partner rather than as a rescuer or a permanent crisis manager. You can stay warm and involved without carrying responsibilities that were never yours to carry. You can protect your own sleep, friendships, work, and interests and still be a good partner, in fact a better one. None of this requires you to love less. It requires you to love from a clearer position.

This book will not teach you to treat post-traumatic stress. That work belongs to trained professionals, and one of the healthiest moves you can make is to stop trying to do it yourself. What this book offers is a way to sort out which parts of the situation are actually yours. The organizing idea runs through every chapter, and it is simple enough to hold in your head during a hard moment. Some things are yours. Some things are your partner's. Some things belong to the relationship, to the two of you together. Yours, theirs, ours. Most of the exhaustion supporting partners feel comes from carrying items that belong in the other two columns. Most of the recovery comes from putting them back.

There is good reason to take the supporting partner seriously, and it is not selfishness. Research on couples affected by trauma describes how one person's symptoms ripple into the other's wellbeing, and how the relationship itself becomes part of the picture rather than a neutral backdrop (Nelson Goff & Smith, 2005). Studies also describe a specific pattern in which partners rearrange their own lives around the symptoms, taking over tasks, avoiding certain topics, canceling plans, walking on eggshells, in ways that are meant to help but that can quietly keep the trauma in place (Fredman et al., 2014). Understanding that pattern, and learning to change it, is a large part of what follows.

A word about what this book is careful not to do. It does not treat your partner as a burden or a problem to be solved. People with trauma histories are not broken objects, and many of them are responsible, capable, loving people who work hard at their own recovery. This book also does not treat every act of caring as a symptom of something wrong with you. Supporting a partner through a hard season is one of the good things human beings do for each other. The aim is not to make you cooler or more detached. The aim is to help you tell the difference between support that keeps love alive and over-functioning that slowly drains it, and to give you specific, workable ways to shift from the second to the first.

The road ahead runs in a deliberate order. The early chapters help you see clearly: how support drifts into a job, and how three very different roles, partner, peer supporter, and clinician, keep getting collapsed into one. The middle chapters give you tools: how to help without taking over, how to set boundaries that are about your own behavior rather than control, and how to survive the guilt that shows up after you finally say no. Later chapters turn outward: how to talk about professional help without becoming the help, how to bring affection and friendship and ordinary life back into a relationship that has narrowed down to symptom management, and how to build real support for yourself. The final chapter draws a line that matters more than any other. Understanding why a person behaves as they do is not the same as accepting behavior that is unsafe, and love never requires you to live in danger.

You do not have to read straight through, though the first two chapters will make the rest easier. Take it at the pace of a real life, not a syllabus. Somewhere in these pages is the version of you who loves this person and still has a self left over. That version is not gone. Let us go find them.

Chapter 1: When Love Quietly Becomes a Job

Solenne is at a dinner party, and she is not really at the dinner party. She is watching Auren. He is three seats away, telling a story about their dog, and to everyone else he looks relaxed. Solenne can see the small signs that no one else reads. The way his thumb is moving against his glass. The way his eyes went to the door when the neighbor's car backfired outside. She has already decided that if the conversation turns to the news, she will change the subject. She has already worked out how to get them home early without it seeming like her idea. She laughs at the right moments and passes the bread and keeps up her half of a conversation about someone's kitchen renovation, and the entire time, a second job is running underneath the first one. When they finally get to the car, Auren says the evening was nice, and it was. He has no idea that Solenne spent it working.

That second job has a name, even if Solenne has never used it. Sociologists call it emotional labor, the effort of managing feelings, yours and other people's, as a kind of unpaid work (Hochschild, 1983). Everyone does some of it. Partners of people with trauma histories often do an enormous amount of it, continuously, and without anyone noticing, including themselves. This chapter is about noticing. Before you can change the role you have taken on, you have to be able to see it, and the strange thing about this particular role is how well it hides.

The yes that never happened

Ask supporting partners when they agreed to become the manager of the household's emotional weather, and you will get a blank look. No one agreed. That is the heart of it. The role arrives through a long series of small, loving decisions, each one reasonable on its own. Your partner has a bad night, so you handle the morning. They cannot face a phone call, so you make it. A certain restaurant is hard for them, so you stop suggesting it. None of these choices is a mistake. Added together over months and years, they become a job description you never applied for.

I call the place where care turns into management the drift line, because you do not cross it in a single step. You drift across it. On one side, you are a partner doing kind things for someone you love. On the other side, you are running a person's life for them, tracking their moods like a weather service, and quietly organizing the world so that nothing difficult ever reaches them. The two sides can look almost identical from the outside. The difference is not how much you do. The difference is who the doing belongs to and what it is teaching both of you.

The Drift Line. Support becomes a job by slow drift, not by decision. You can learn to find the line where caring for your partner turned into managing them, and most of what exhausts you lives on the far side of that line.

What the research actually shows

There is a temptation, when you first see this pattern in yourself, to feel foolish, as if you should have known better. You should not. The pattern is well documented, and it is not a sign of weakness or poor judgment. Researchers who study couples affected by trauma describe how one partner's symptoms move through the relationship and shape the other partner's inner life, so that trauma stops being one person's problem and becomes a shared system (Nelson Goff & Smith, 2005). You are not imagining the pull. It is real, and it is strong.

More specifically, clinicians have a term for the set of behaviors Solenne was doing at that dinner. They call it accommodation. Accommodation includes avoiding topics that might upset your partner, taking over tasks they find hard, canceling plans to spare them a difficult situation, and adjusting your own behavior to prevent an angry or anxious reaction (Fredman et al., 2014). Read that list again. Every item is something a loving person does. And here is the part that matters. When researchers followed couples over time, higher levels of this accommodation were linked to more distress in the supporting partner and, in some cases, to the trauma symptoms holding steady rather than easing (Fredman et al., 2022). The very behaviors meant to protect your partner can help keep them stuck, because the world never asks them to do the hard thing, so the hard thing never gets less hard.

Sit with that, because it reframes the whole situation. Your exhaustion is not the price of being a good partner. Some of it is the price of doing a job that does not work, a job that costs you a great deal and gives your partner less than you hoped. That is not a reason for guilt. It is a reason for a different plan.

The monitor never clocks out

Consider Vaelan, thirty-nine, whose wife Aeris survived a violent robbery two years ago. Aeris is doing the real work of recovery. She has a therapist she trusts and she is, most weeks, moving forward. Vaelan is proud of her. He is also, by his own description, tired all the way to his bones, and he cannot explain why, because on paper he is not doing much. He is not the one with nightmares. He is not the one who flinches at a stranger's raised voice.

What Vaelan is doing is monitoring. From the moment he wakes, part of his attention is on Aeris. How did she sleep. What is her face doing. Is today a good day or a bad day, and which version of the evening should he prepare for. He scans her the way a lifeguard scans a pool, and like a lifeguard, he never fully relaxes, because the whole point is to catch the danger before it happens. The monitoring is invisible. No one sees it, so no one credits it, and Vaelan himself dismisses it, telling himself he is not really doing anything. But vigilance is work, some of the most tiring work there is, and a mind that is always half on someone else is a mind that never rests.

This is worth naming clearly, because supporting partners routinely undercount their own effort. They compare their fatigue to their partner's obvious struggle, decide they have no right to be tired, and push the fatigue down. The monitoring does not stop. It just goes unacknowledged, which is the worst of both worlds. You pay the cost and deny yourself the credit.

Try this week: the monitor's inventory. For three days, keep a note, on your phone or a scrap of paper, of every moment you catch yourself scanning your partner or adjusting your behavior to manage their state. You are not trying to stop yet. You are only counting. Note the time and one or two words: "checked her face at breakfast," "changed the subject away from the news," "canceled seeing Dad so he wouldn't have to." At the end of three days, read the list. Most people are startled by its length. That list is the job you never applied for, written out at last.

Three columns, one relationship

The rest of this book turns on a single distinction, and this is the place to introduce it. In any relationship touched by trauma, the responsibilities fall into three groups. Some belong to you. Your sleep, your friendships, your work, your health, your reactions, your choices. Some belong to your partner. Their recovery, their appointments, their feelings, their symptoms, the daily work of managing their own condition. And some belong to the relationship itself, to the two of you together. The chores, the money, the plans, the affection, the way you treat each other, the shared dreams. Yours, theirs, ours.

Almost all of the drift you have been reading about is the drift of items out of the "theirs" column and into the "yours" column. Your partner's phone calls become your phone calls. Your partner's difficult feelings become your responsibility to prevent. Your partner's recovery becomes a project you manage. Each transfer feels like love, and some transfers, in a hard week, genuinely are. The problem is that they rarely transfer back. The columns get lopsided, and a lopsided arrangement, held for years, is what burnout is made of.

You do not have to sort every item today. For now, it is enough to hold the three columns in mind and to notice that the question "whose is this, really" has a real answer more often than you think. When the toddler-level tiredness hits at the end of a day when nothing dramatic happened, it is usually because you spent the day carrying things from the wrong column.

Try this week: the three-column glance. Take five items from your monitor's inventory. For each one, ask the plain question: is this mine, is it theirs, or is it ours. Do not decide what to do about any of them. Just write the letter next to each: M, T, or O. Notice how many landed as T, things that are genuinely your partner's, that you have been carrying anyway. That noticing is the whole exercise. The doing comes later.

Why seeing it feels like grief

There is a reaction that often comes when a supporting partner first sees the drift line clearly, and it is not relief. It is something closer to grief, and it is worth preparing for. When you realize how much you have been carrying, you may also realize how long you have been carrying it, and how much of yourself you set down along the way. The evenings with friends you stopped accepting. The hobby that quietly ended. The version of your marriage you thought you were signing up for. Seeing the job means seeing its cost, and the cost can be large.

Let that reaction come. Do not rush past it into problem-solving, and do not talk yourself out of it by comparing your loss to your partner's trauma, as if only one of you is allowed to have lost something. Two things are true at once. Your partner survived something terrible and deserves support. And you gave up real parts of your life, often without deciding to, and those parts mattered. Holding both of those truths, without letting either one cancel the other, is the emotional skill this whole book asks you to build. It starts here, with letting yourself feel the weight of a job you can finally see.

Solenne did this exercise, the monitor's inventory, over a long weekend. She stopped counting at forty items and cried in the car outside a grocery store, not because anything was wrong that day, but because the list was so long and so invisible and so entirely uncredited. Then she dried her face and drove home and did not, that week, change anything at all. That was fine. Seeing the job clearly, and grieving it a little, was the work of that week. She was not behind. She was exactly where the first real step is.

The story you tell about the tiredness

There is one more thing to notice this week, and it lives not in your behavior but in the story you tell yourself about it. When supporting partners finally admit how tired they are, they usually reach for an explanation that blames themselves. I must be weak. I must not love them enough, or I would not resent this. Other people manage, so something is wrong with me. That story is false, and it is expensive, because it adds shame to exhaustion and shame is heavy in its own right.

The accurate story is different and kinder without being soft. You are tired because you have been doing a large, invisible, unshared job for a long time, a job that would tire anyone, and the fact that you are tired is evidence of how much you have carried, not evidence of any defect in you. Vaelan spent two years convinced he was simply not a strong enough person, comparing himself to some imagined partner who would find all this effortless. When he understood that vigilance is genuine work and that no one does it without cost, the shame lifted, and the strange thing was that lifting the shame gave him more energy, not less. Shame is a tax on effort. Dropping the false story is like getting a refund.

This matters practically, because the story you tell shapes what you allow yourself to do next. If your tiredness means you are weak, then the only honorable response is to try harder, which is exactly the wrong direction. If your tiredness means you have been carrying too much, then the honorable response is to set some of it down, which is the direction this whole book runs. The story is not a small thing. It is the difference between a supporter who pushes toward burnout and one who begins, at last, to redistribute the load.

Try this week: catch the false story. When you notice the tiredness this week, listen for the explanation your mind offers. If it blames you, weak, selfish, not loving enough, write down the accurate version instead: "I am tired because I have carried a heavy, invisible job for a long time, and that would tire anyone." You do not have to believe it fully yet. You only have to write it down next to the false one, so you can see that there is a choice about which story to keep.

There is a reason this book starts here, with seeing rather than doing. Every technique in the chapters ahead depends on your being able to tell, in a given moment, whether an act is support or management, whether a task is yours or someone else's, whether a feeling is a fact or just a feeling. That discernment begins with the plain act of noticing, which is why your only assignments this week are to count and to look. You are building the eyes you will need for everything that follows, and eyes take a little time to adjust to a room you have been sitting in, in the dark, for years.

The through-line

You did not choose this role, but you can choose what happens next, and the first choice is simply to see it plainly. Support drifts into management one small yes at a time, until a loving partner is also running a person's life and calling the exhaustion normal. The three columns give you a way to sort the load, and the monitor's inventory gives you a way to see it. None of that requires you to love your partner less, and none of it makes their trauma less real. It only asks you to stop pretending the job is not a job.

In the next chapter we sharpen the picture. Much of the drift you just uncovered comes from a specific confusion, the collapsing of three very different roles into one overworked person. There is the partner, the peer who supports, and the professional who treats. You have been asked, or have asked yourself, to be all three at once. It cannot be done, and the attempt is quietly breaking you. It is time to pull those roles apart.

Chapter 2: Partner, Supporter, Clinician: Different Roles

Isoren found the worksheet in a drawer while looking for tape. It was a trigger log, the kind a therapist gives a client, with columns for the situation, the feeling, the body sensation, the thought. Isoren had filled it in. Not Cyrel, the person in therapy. Isoren, the partner. At some point over the past year, Isoren had started keeping notes on Cyrel's reactions, tracking patterns, and gently walking Cyrel through them at the kitchen table on bad evenings. "It sounds like that was a flashback, love. Remember what happens in your nervous system when." Isoren had read three books on complex trauma and could explain the window of tolerance better than some professionals. And Cyrel, forty, who lives with complex post-traumatic stress from a childhood no child should survive, was not getting better. If anything, the two of them were more tangled and more tired than they had been a year ago.

Isoren was doing a good and loving thing in the wrong chair. That is what this chapter is about. In any relationship touched by trauma, there are three roles that people confuse constantly, because from the outside they can look like the same warm act of caring. There is the partner. There is the peer who supports. And there is the professional who treats. They are not interchangeable, and one person cannot hold all three at once without harm to everyone involved.

Three chairs, not one

Imagine three chairs in a room. In the first chair sits the partner. The partner's job is intimacy: to love, to share a life, to be a companion and a lover and a teammate, to know the person and be known by them. In the second chair sits the peer supporter, the friend or family member who offers encouragement, a listening ear, practical help, and steady company through a hard time. In the third chair sits the clinician, the trained professional who assesses, treats, and takes responsibility for the technical work of recovery.

You can move between the first two chairs fairly naturally. Partners support their partners, and supporters can be intimate with the people they support. But the third chair is different. It requires training, a professional frame, and a deliberate distance that is the opposite of intimacy. A therapist does not share your bed, depend on you for rent, or feel their own night ruined when the session goes badly. That distance is not coldness. It is part of what makes the treatment work. When you try to sit in the third chair while also sitting in the first, you get neither a good therapist nor a whole partner. You get an exhausted person doing two jobs badly and slowly losing the relationship that made them want to help in the first place.

The Third Chair. Intimacy, peer support, and professional treatment are three different chairs. You can move between the first two, but you cannot sit in the clinician's chair and the partner's chair at the same time, and every attempt to do so costs you both.

What complex trauma actually asks for

To see why the clinician's chair is not yours to take, it helps to understand a little about what Cyrel is dealing with. Complex trauma, which grows out of prolonged and repeated harm, often in childhood and often at the hands of people who were supposed to provide care, is not the same as a single terrible event. The psychiatrist Judith Herman, who first described this pattern, noted that it affects a person's sense of safety, their relationships, and their very sense of self, not just their memory of what happened (Herman, 2015). The World Health Organization now recognizes complex post-traumatic stress disorder as a distinct condition, adding difficulties with emotion regulation, self-worth, and relationships to the core features of ordinary post-traumatic stress (World Health Organization, 2019).

Notice what that means. The wound is, in large part, a wound in relationships. That is exactly why an intimate partner cannot be the one to treat it, and also why an intimate partner matters so much. The relationship is where the injury shows up most, which makes you a powerful source of safety and also the least suited person to run the clinical repair. A skilled clinician can hold steady when Cyrel's trauma reaches out and tests whether this person, too, will hurt or abandon him. You cannot hold that steadiness, because you are not neutral. You are the person he loves and fears losing, which is precisely what makes you unable to be his therapist. That is not a failing. It is the nature of love.

What a partner can actually do

If the clinician's chair is off limits, it is fair to ask what is left. A great deal, as it turns out, and most of it is more useful than amateur therapy. A partner can offer safety, the ordinary, daily kind: predictability, warmth, a home that is not another source of threat. A partner can offer company that is not about trauma at all, which matters more than it sounds, because a person reduced to their diagnosis loses track of the rest of who they are. A partner can support the treatment without becoming it, by making space for appointments, by not undermining the work, by being someone the person can come home to. And a partner can share a life: cook dinner, argue about the thermostat, laugh at a bad movie, want each other. That list is not a consolation prize. It is the actual relationship, the thing that both of you presumably want to protect.

What a partner is not equipped to do is assess symptoms, guide exposure work, reframe cognitive distortions on the fly, or take responsibility for the direction of someone's recovery. When Isoren walked Cyrel through his flashback at the kitchen table, Isoren was doing clinical work without clinical training, without a professional frame, and without the ability to step back at the end of the hour. It felt like intimacy. It was actually a slow erosion of intimacy, because every evening turned into a session, and a marriage cannot survive on sessions.

The cost of the collapsed role

When the three chairs collapse into one, specific things break, and they break in predictable ways. The partner loses the relationship, because there is no longer any time when they are simply together rather than working. The person with trauma loses a refuge, because home becomes another clinical setting, and there is nowhere that is not about their condition. And the recovery itself can stall, because homemade therapy delivered by an emotionally involved partner is not as effective as the real thing, and it can crowd out the professional help that would actually move things forward.

There is also a subtler cost, and Isoren felt it without being able to name it. Resentment. When you take on a role that is too big for anyone, part of you keeps score, even if you would never say so out loud. You gave up your evenings, your patience, your own inner life, and some quiet part of you begins to feel owed. That resentment is not a character flaw. It is the natural result of doing an impossible job. It is also poison to intimacy, because it lives in the same body that is supposed to feel affection, and the two cannot occupy the same space for long.

Try this week: which chair am I in. For one week, when you catch yourself in a caring moment with your partner, pause and ask which chair you are sitting in. Partner, supporter, or clinician. You are not judging yourself. You are locating yourself. If you are explaining their nervous system to them, interpreting their symptoms, running an exercise you read about, or trying to produce a therapeutic outcome, you are in the third chair. Simply notice, and if you can, gently return to the first chair by doing something ordinary instead: make tea, hold their hand, say "that sounds hard," and stop there.

Stopping there is the skill

That last instruction deserves its own attention, because "stop there" is the hardest sentence in this chapter. When your partner is in pain, every instinct pushes you to do more, to fix, to explain, to resolve. Stopping after "that sounds hard" can feel like abandoning them mid-sentence. It is not. It is the difference between the second chair and the third. A peer supporter listens, cares, and stays present without trying to run the treatment. A clinician does the treatment. You can be the first. You cannot, and should not, be the last.

Isoren tried this for a week and found it almost unbearable at first. On the third evening, Cyrel came home shaking after a hard day, and every part of Isoren wanted to reach for the trigger log, to name what was happening, to guide him through it. Instead Isoren made soup, sat close, and said, "I'm here. You don't have to explain it to me." Cyrel cried, and then, after a while, he stopped, and they ate soup. Nothing was cured. But for the first time in a long time, the kitchen was a kitchen and not a clinic, and both of them slept a little better.

When you slide back

You will slide back into the clinician's chair. Everyone does, especially at first, because the pull to fix a beloved person's pain is one of the strongest pulls there is. Sliding back is not failure. The skill is noticing you have done it and climbing out again, without a long detour into self-criticism. Isoren still slips, still sometimes starts analyzing Cyrel's reactions before catching it. The difference now is the catching. The average has shifted. Home is a clinic less often than it used to be, and the marriage has a little more room to breathe.

Try this week: the job description you decline. Write a short list titled "Not my job." On it, put the specific clinical tasks you have been quietly doing: interpreting their symptoms, guiding exposure, tracking their triggers, managing their medication, being the one who processes every flashback. You are not declining to care. You are declining to do the professional's work. Keep the list where you can see it, and when you feel yourself drifting toward the third chair, read it. Some things are theirs, and some things belong to a trained person who is not you.

Telling your partner about the chairs

At some point you may want to explain this shift to your partner, because if you quietly stop doing homemade therapy without a word, your partner may experience it as withdrawal rather than repair. The conversation is delicate, and it goes best when it is framed as a change in you rather than a complaint about them. The message is not "you have been using me as your therapist." The message is "I have realized I have been trying to be your therapist, and I am not good at it, and it has been crowding out the part of us that I love most."

Framed that way, the conversation is an invitation rather than an accusation. You can say that you want to go back to being their partner, their companion, the person they come home to, rather than the person running their treatment. You can say that this does not mean you care less, and that you will still be beside them, listening and supporting, just not trying to do the professional's job at the kitchen table. Many partners, told this, feel relief rather than rejection, because home has become a clinic for them too, and they miss the ordinary relationship as much as you do.

Isoren had this conversation with Cyrel after a few weeks of quietly staying out of the clinician's chair. Cyrel had noticed the change and, for a moment, feared it meant Isoren was pulling away, giving up on him. When Isoren explained the three chairs and said, "I want to be your partner again, not your therapist, because I love being your partner and I was terrible at being your therapist," Cyrel laughed for the first time in what felt like weeks. He had felt the clinic-ification of their home as keenly as Isoren had. Naming it out loud let them both set it down together.

Not every partner responds this well, and some will need reassurance more than once that stepping out of the clinician's chair is not the same as stepping out of the relationship. That reassurance is worth giving, patiently, because the distinction is real and important, and your partner may have to hear it several times before they trust it. What you are offering is not less love. It is love in its proper chair.

It helps to remember that the roles are not ranked. The partner is not a lesser thing than the clinician, and stepping out of the third chair is not a demotion. If anything, the partner's chair is the one no professional can ever fill, the chair of the person who shares your life and loves you across years. A therapist, however skilled, goes home at the end of the hour to their own life. You are the home your partner comes back to. That is not a smaller role than the clinician's. It is a different one, and a rarer one, and it is worth protecting from the slow encroachment of a job that was never yours.

You may worry that pulling the roles apart will leave your partner feeling unsupported, as though you are withdrawing something they depend on. In practice the opposite tends to happen. When you stop trying to be the clinician, you usually become a better partner and a better peer supporter, because you are no longer stretched across three jobs and quietly resentful of all of them. Your listening improves when it is not secretly an assessment. Your comfort lands more warmly when it is not the opening move of a treatment plan. What your partner loses is amateur therapy they were not benefiting from anyway. What they gain is more of the real you.

The through-line

The exhaustion you named in the first chapter has a specific engine, and this chapter has shown it to you. You have been trying to sit in three chairs at once, and the clinician's chair, in particular, was never yours to occupy. Pulling the roles apart does not make you a worse partner. It makes you a real one, freed from a job that was breaking you and, quietly, keeping your partner stuck. The relationship gets its evenings back. The recovery gets a professional. And you get to be the person your partner loves rather than the person managing their condition.

Understanding the roles, though, is not the same as escaping the pull that keeps dragging you into the wrong one. In the next chapter we look closely at that pull, the specific loop of fear, guilt, crisis, and momentary relief that keeps yanking supporting partners back into over-functioning even after they know better. It is called the rescue loop, and once you can see its mechanics, you can start to step out of it.

Chapter 3: The Rescue Loop

The text came at 11:40 on a Tuesday night. Lysant was already in bed. Sevrin, her husband, was still up, and the message read: "I can't do the meeting tomorrow. I can't. Can you call them." Lysant felt the familiar drop in her stomach, the one that arrives whenever Sevrin is in distress, and within a minute she was out of bed, at her laptop, drafting an email to his manager explaining that Sevrin was unwell and would need to reschedule. She sent it at midnight. Sevrin's whole body loosened. He thanked her, held her, fell asleep almost at once. Lysant lay awake for another hour, wired and vaguely sick, telling herself she had done the right thing. In the morning, Sevrin was calmer than he had been in days, and Lysant took that as proof. It was proof, but not of what she thought.

What happened that night was not simply a kind act. It was one full turn of a loop, and the loop is the reason supporting partners keep over-functioning long after they know it is hurting them. Understanding the loop is the difference between a pattern that runs you and a pattern you can interrupt. This chapter takes it apart, gear by gear.

Four gears, turning fast

The rescue loop has four parts, and it turns quickly, often in minutes. First comes the trigger: your partner's distress, or the threat of it. Second comes your fear, which may not feel like fear. It may feel like urgency, or love, or simple certainty that you must act now. Third comes the rescue: you step in and take over the hard thing, whatever it is. And fourth comes relief, for both of you. Your partner's distress drops, and so does yours, because their calm is what you were after all along.

That fourth gear is the trap. The relief feels like evidence that you did the right thing, and it teaches your brain a lesson: rescuing works. It makes the bad feeling go away. So the next time the trigger comes, the pull to rescue is a little stronger, because it has been rewarded. This is one of the most reliable ways any behavior gets locked in. When an action removes something unpleasant, we do it more, and we do it faster, and we stop questioning it. The loop does not survive because you are weak. It survives because it works in the short term, every single time.

The Relief Trap. The momentary relief you feel after rescuing your partner is exactly what teaches you to rescue again. Short-term calm quietly buys long-term over-functioning, and the better the relief feels, the tighter the trap.

What relief hides

Here is what the relief hides. That night, Lysant did not just calm Sevrin. She also made sure that Sevrin never had to make the hard phone call himself, never had to sit with his own discomfort, never got the chance to discover that he could survive a difficult conversation with his manager. The meeting stayed frightening, because he never approached it. And a lesson was reinforced on his side too: when things get hard, Lysant handles it.

This is not a story about a manipulative partner. Sevrin was not scheming. He was in real distress and reached for the person who always helps. That is the ordinary tragedy of the loop. Two people who love each other build, without meaning to, a system in which one person's world keeps shrinking and the other person's load keeps growing, and both of them mistake it for devotion. Researchers have watched this happen in careful studies. When partners accommodate trauma symptoms on a given day, taking over, smoothing the path, removing the obstacle, the person with trauma tends to show more avoidance the next day, not less (Allen et al., 2021; Fredman et al., 2022). The rescue does not resolve the fear. It feeds it.

Why you do it, really

It is worth being clear-eyed about the reasons you rescue, because they are not all the same, and some are riskier than others. When researchers asked partners why they accommodate, the most common reasons were a sense of obligation and a wish to protect the relationship (Renshaw et al., 2020). Those are decent, human reasons. But the study found something important. Partners who accommodated mainly out of conflict avoidance and helplessness, a sense of "I just don't know what else to do, and I can't stand the fight," tended to have the worst outcomes, more distress and lower satisfaction (Renshaw et al., 2020). The reason behind the rescue matters. Rescuing because you briefly cannot tolerate your own fear is different from rescuing after a clear-eyed decision that this particular help is worth giving.

That distinction gives you a tool. The next time you feel the pull to rescue, you can ask: am I doing this because it is genuinely the right support, or am I doing it to make my own fear stop. Both feel identical in the moment. Only one of them is a decision. The other is the loop, wearing the mask of love.

Support and rescue are not the same

People often hear all this and swing to the opposite extreme, deciding they must never help with anything, which is its own kind of mistake. The goal is not to stop supporting your partner. The goal is to tell support and rescue apart, because they are genuinely different, even when they look alike.

Support keeps the responsibility with your partner while offering help. Rescue takes the responsibility away. Support might sound like, "That call sounds really hard. Do you want to think through what you'd say, or would it help if I sat with you while you make it." Rescue sounds like, "Don't worry, I'll do it." Support leaves your partner standing, with you beside them. Rescue picks them up and carries them, which feels tender and, done constantly, teaches them they cannot walk. One occasional carry, in a genuine crisis, is fine and human. A relationship built on carrying is the thing that breaks you both.

Consider Novaire, fifty-two, whose partner Lorien has post-traumatic stress after a serious workplace accident. For two years Novaire rescued constantly, and both of them were miserable. When she learned to distinguish support from rescue, she did not become cold. She changed the shape of her help. When Lorien froze before a medical appointment, she stopped canceling it for him. Instead she said, "I'll drive you and wait in the car, but the appointment is yours." The first time, Lorien was furious and frightened, and it was an awful morning. He also went in. It did not fix everything, and there were later mornings when the old pattern won. But something had shifted. Lorien had proof that he could do a hard thing with Novaire beside him rather than in front of him, and that proof, unlike rescue, actually reduced the fear over time.

Catching the loop mid-turn

You cannot interrupt a loop you cannot see, so the first skill is simply to catch it turning. The clearest place to catch it is at the fourth gear, the relief, because that is where the trap closes. After you rescue and feel the flood of relief, that is your signal. Not a signal that you did wrong, but a signal that the loop just completed a turn. Noticing the relief, and naming it privately as "that was the loop, not a verdict," starts to loosen its grip.

Try this week: map one turn of the loop. Think of a recent time you stepped in to handle something for your partner. On paper, write the four gears. What was the trigger. What did you feel, and was it urgency or fear underneath. What did you do. And what was the relief, for each of you. Then add one more line: what did your partner not get the chance to do because you did it for them. That last line is not to make you feel guilty. It is to make the loop visible, so that next time you can see it coming.

The twenty-four-hour experiment

Once you can see the loop, you can begin to slow it down, and speed is the loop's main weapon. It turns so fast that there is no gap for a decision. The remedy is to build a gap.

Try this week: the pause before the rescue. The next time a non-emergency request to rescue arrives, and only when there is no genuine safety issue, try inserting a pause before you act. It can be short. "Let me think about the best way to help with that, and let's talk in the morning."

Then notice what happens in the gap. Often your own fear peaks and then falls on its own, and you discover the situation was not as urgent as it felt. Sometimes your partner, given a little space, handles part of it themselves. And sometimes, after the pause, you decide the help is worth giving, and you give it, now as a choice rather than a reflex. The pause does not make you unkind. It converts the loop back into a relationship, where both people get to think.

Lysant tried the pause a week after that midnight email. Sevrin asked her, again late at night, to handle something that could wait. This time she said, "I love you, and I want to help. Let's figure it out tomorrow when we're both thinking straight." She did not sleep easily that first night either, because the fear does not vanish just because you named it. But she noticed, in the morning, that the world had not ended, and that Sevrin had actually drafted part of the thing himself before she woke. It was one small turn of the loop, left uncompleted. That is how the loop loosens. Not all at once, but one uncompleted turn at a time.

Real emergencies are different

A caution is needed here, because a reader can take the idea of the rescue loop too far and decide never to step in for anything, which is neither safe nor loving. Some situations are genuine emergencies, and in a genuine emergency you should act, fully and without a twenty-four-hour pause. The skill is not to stop helping. It is to tell a real emergency apart from the manufactured urgency the loop generates, because the loop dresses every request in the costume of a crisis.

A real emergency involves genuine, immediate risk to safety, health, or something that truly cannot wait, and it is relatively rare. Manufactured urgency involves ordinary difficulty that feels unbearable in the moment and demands to be solved right now, and it is common. The tell is often in your own body. Manufactured urgency comes with that frantic, must-fix-it-now pressure that will not tolerate a pause. Real emergencies, oddly, sometimes come with a colder clarity. When you learn to notice the frantic pressure and recognize it as the loop rather than as accurate information about the stakes, you can pause on the manufactured ones and act on the real ones, instead of treating everything as a five alarm fire.

There is also a middle category worth naming: things that are important but not emergencies. A missed deadline, a hard conversation, a difficult appointment. These feel urgent and are not, and they are exactly where support, rather than rescue, belongs. You do not have to solve them instantly, and you do not have to ignore them either. You can help with them as a partner beside your partner, at a human pace, which is different from either dropping everything to rescue or coldly refusing to engage.

Lysant learned, over time, to sort her late-night texts into these categories. Most were manufactured urgency, and she learned to pause on them. A few were genuine emergencies, and she acted on those without hesitation and without guilt. The sorting itself, the moment of asking "is this actually an emergency, or is this the loop," was what gave her back some control. She was no longer at the mercy of every wave of urgency. She was making decisions again, which is the opposite of what the loop had trained her to do.

One more thing about the loop, because it explains a puzzle many supporting partners feel. You may have noticed that the more you rescue, the more rescuing seems to be required, as if your help were making the need grow rather than shrink. You are not imagining it, and you are not doing it wrong. That is simply what the loop does. Each rescue teaches your partner that the hard thing gets handled by you, and teaches you that handling it makes the fear stop, so both of you reach for the pattern more readily next time. The escalation is not a sign that your partner is getting worse or that you are failing. It is the loop doing exactly what loops do, and seeing that clearly is the first thing that lets you step out of it rather than pedaling harder inside it.

It is also worth forgiving yourself for how long the loop has run. Supporting partners often feel foolish once they see the pattern, as though they should have caught it years ago. But the loop is designed, by its very structure, to be invisible, because every single turn is rewarded and every reward feels like love. You were not being naive. You were being human, responding to relief the way all humans respond to relief. Seeing the loop at all puts you ahead of where most people ever get, and the seeing is what matters now, not the years it took to see. Blame added on top of the loop only makes it heavier. Set it down and start counting turns, because the counting, not the blame, is what finally slows the loop enough for a real decision to fit inside it.

The through-line

The rescue loop keeps you over-functioning because it pays you, in relief, every time you obey it, while quietly charging your partner's recovery and your own reserves the real cost. Its four gears turn fast, but they can be slowed. When you can name the relief as the trap rather than the reward, tell support apart from rescue, and build a pause into the moment before you act, the loop stops running you. You begin to choose your help instead of reflexively delivering it.

Choosing your help, though, raises a harder question. If you are not going to rescue, what do you do instead when your partner is struggling and you want to be useful. The answer is not to stand back and do nothing. It is to help in a way that keeps your partner in the driver's seat of their own life. In the next chapter we look at exactly how to do that: how to replace fixing with questions, choices, and shared responsibility, so that helping stops meaning taking over.

Chapter 4: Helping Without Taking Over

Auren mentioned, one evening, that he had gotten a letter from the veterans' benefits office and did not understand it. Solenne, who has read this book's earlier chapters in her own life if not on paper, felt the old pull to take the letter, decode it, make the calls, and hand him back a solved problem. She had done exactly that a hundred times. This time she sat on her hands, metaphorically, and asked a question instead. "Do you want me to take care of it, or do you want to work through it together, or do you want to handle it yourself and just talk it out with me first." Auren was quiet for a moment, surprised to be asked. Then he said, "Together, I think. I don't want to do it alone, but I don't want you doing it for me either." They spread the letter on the table and read it side by side. It took longer than if Solenne had done it herself. It was also the first time in months that Auren had faced a piece of official paper without either panicking or disappearing, and he ended the evening looking, if not proud, then at least less small.

That question Solenne asked is the whole subject of this chapter. When you decide to stop rescuing, a gap opens, and the gap frightens people, because it feels like the only alternative to taking over is doing nothing. There is a third option, and it is where good support actually lives. You can help in a way that keeps your partner in charge of their own life. The name for it, in the research, is autonomy support, and it is one of the most useful ideas a supporting partner can learn.

The urge to fix has a name

There is a specific reflex that drives most over-helping, and naming it helps you resist it. Clinicians who study behavior change call it the righting reflex, the almost irresistible urge to set things right for a struggling person, to jump in and fix the problem you can plainly see (Miller & Rollnick, 2013). The reflex comes from a good place. You care, you can see the solution, and it seems obvious that you should provide it. But when you fix a problem for someone who could, with support, have faced it themselves, you send a quiet message: I don't think you are capable of handling this. Do that often enough and the person starts to believe it.

The counterintuitive finding is that people change and grow best when their sense of choice is protected rather than overridden. Human beings have a basic need to feel that their actions are their own, and when that need is met, their motivation is stronger and their wellbeing is higher (Deci & Ryan, 2000). When it is not met, when someone is constantly directed, managed, and done-for, motivation drains away, even when the directing is loving. Your partner's recovery runs on their own motivation. Every time you take the wheel, you are, with the kindest intentions, siphoning off the fuel.

Hands Off the Wheel. Help that removes your partner's choices also removes their recovery. You can sit in the passenger seat and be endlessly useful, but the moment you grab the wheel, you take something from them that no amount of caring gives back.

Ask before you help

The simplest tool in this chapter is also the one supporting partners resist most, because it feels almost too small to matter. Ask before you help. Instead of assuming you know what your partner needs and delivering it, ask them what kind of help, if any, they want.

This matters because the help you would choose is often not the help they need, and delivering the wrong help, insistently, is its own burden. Sometimes a person wants a solution. Sometimes they only want to be heard and would find your solution intrusive. Sometimes they want to do it themselves and simply need you nearby. You cannot know which without asking, and asking does something beyond getting the answer right. It hands your partner the dignity of choosing, which is exactly the thing trauma so often strips away.

Try this week: the help question. When your partner is struggling with something concrete, resist the reflex to jump in. Instead, ask a version of the question Solenne asked: "Do you want me to handle it, do you want to do it together, or do you want to do it yourself and talk it through with me." Then honor the answer, even if it is not the one you would have picked. If they choose to do it themselves and it goes imperfectly, let it. An imperfect thing they did is worth more, for their recovery, than a perfect thing you did for them.

Offer choices, not verdicts

When help is genuinely wanted, there is a way to give it that adds to your partner's sense of agency rather than subtracting from it. Offer options instead of instructions. "You could call them, or you could email, or you could ask your therapist to help you plan it. What feels most possible right now." This is not a trick to get them to do what you want. It is a real handing-over of choice. The difference between "here is what you should do" and "here are some ways you could go, and you decide" is small in words and large in effect. The first is a verdict delivered from above. The second treats your partner as the competent adult they are, even on a day when they do not feel like one.

Consider Éloane, thirty-one, whose partner Zevian struggles with severe anxiety following a traumatic loss. Éloane used to plan Zevian's days for him, deciding when he should rest, what he should eat, whether he was ready to see people. It came from love and it left Zevian feeling like a patient in his own home. When Éloane switched from directing to offering, the change was not instant, and there were arguments about it, because Zevian had grown used to being managed and part of him resented being handed responsibility he did not always want. But over months, Zevian began making more of his own small choices, and a few of the choices Éloane would never have picked turned out to be exactly what he needed. Éloane had to tolerate getting it "wrong" by her own standards. That tolerance was the price of Zevian getting himself back.

Shared responsibility, not transferred responsibility

The three columns from the first chapter return here in a practical form. When something needs doing, the reflexive move is to transfer it entirely into your column: I'll do it, don't worry about it. The healthier move is often to keep it shared, in the "ours" column, or to keep it in theirs while you support from the side. Shared responsibility means you both have a part, and neither part is "carry the whole thing."

This looks like specifics. If a bill needs paying and your partner is overwhelmed, shared responsibility might be: you sit together, they enter the numbers while you find the account details. If a hard conversation with a family member is looming, it might be: they decide what to say, you help them rehearse it. In each case, the responsibility stays partly with the person whose life it belongs to. You are not abandoning them. You are refusing to do the one thing that would harm them most, which is to make their life something that happens to them while you run it.

Try this week: split one task. Pick one thing you would normally take over completely for your partner. Instead of doing all of it, split it. Do one part and leave one part for them, chosen together. The split does not have to be even. The point is that your partner keeps a piece of their own life in their own hands, and you resist the urge to swallow the whole task in the name of love.

When they choose not to act

Autonomy support contains a hard truth that rescue never has to face. When you hand your partner the choice, they may choose not to act, and you have to let that be their choice too. This is where supporting partners often panic and grab the wheel back. Auren might decide not to deal with the benefits letter at all. Zevian might choose to stay home when Éloane hoped he would come out. Respecting autonomy means respecting choices you would not make, including the choice to leave something undone.

There are limits, of course. If a choice creates genuine danger, that is a different situation, and we come to it in the final chapter. But for the ordinary hard things, the missed opportunities and the avoided tasks that are frustrating but not dangerous, your job is not to force the outcome. Your job is to offer real support and then let your partner be the author of their own recovery, at their own pace, including the parts of that pace that worry you. You can say, "I think it would help you to do this, and I'll support you if you decide to. And it's yours to decide." Then you have to mean the second sentence, which is the hard part.

The help that builds capacity

There is a simple test you can apply to any act of help, and it clarifies almost every situation. Ask: does this help build my partner's capacity, or replace it. Help that builds capacity leaves your partner more able to face the next thing: they did it, or did part of it, and they have proof they can. Help that replaces capacity leaves them exactly as unable as before, or more so, because you did it and they did not. Both kinds of help feel loving in the moment. Only one of them is on your partner's side over time.

This test cuts through a lot of confusion. Making the phone call for a partner who could, with support, have made it themselves replaces capacity. Sitting beside them while they make it builds capacity. Doing the taxes alone every year because it stresses them replaces capacity. Doing them together, teaching as you go, builds it. You do not have to apply the test perfectly. You only have to start asking the question, and let it tilt your choices, over time, toward the help that leaves your partner stronger.

Try this week: the capacity test. Before you help with something this week, pause and ask whether this particular help builds or replaces your partner's capacity. If it replaces, see whether there is a version that builds instead. You will not always choose the capacity-building version, because some days everyone is too tired, and that is human. But asking the question, even when you override it, keeps you aware of what your help is doing.

Your choices count too

There is a hidden asymmetry in everything this chapter has said, and it is worth dragging into the light. Autonomy support asks you to protect your partner's right to choose. It should also protect yours. Supporting partners become so focused on preserving the other person's agency that they quietly surrender their own, deferring every decision, shaping every plan around the partner's needs, until they are as choiceless as they fear their partner is. That is not balance. It is the same problem wearing the opposite mask.

The three columns cut both ways. Just as some things belong to your partner and should stay theirs, some things belong to you and should stay yours: how you spend an afternoon, whether you see a friend, what you eat, when you rest, what you want for your own future. When you hand those choices over in the name of being a good supporter, you are not being generous. You are erasing yourself, and an erased person cannot support anyone well, because there is no one left to do the supporting.

This is not selfishness, and it is worth insisting on that, because supporting partners are quick to hear any claim on their own life as selfish. A relationship between two people requires two people, both of whom get to want things, choose things, and matter. A relationship in which one person's preferences are the only ones that count is not more loving. It is lopsided, and lopsided arrangements, as we have seen, are where burnout and resentment breed. Protecting your own capacity to choose is part of keeping the relationship a relationship rather than a service you provide.

Éloane discovered this after months of protecting Zevian's autonomy while abandoning her own. She had given Zevian back his choices and, in the process, stopped making any of her own, planning nothing, wanting nothing out loud, treating her own preferences as an imposition.

When she began, cautiously, to name what she wanted, an evening with friends, a say in their plans, a weekend that was partly about her, the relationship did not suffer. It steadied, because Zevian no longer had to carry the strange weight of being the only person in the marriage who was allowed to have needs. Two people choosing is harder than one person deferring. It is also the only version that lasts.

It helps to lower the stakes on getting this right. You will not perfectly balance help and autonomy, and you do not need to. Some days you will take over when you should have stepped back, and some days you will step back when a little more help would have been kinder. Autonomy support is not a test you pass or fail. It is a direction you lean, over hundreds of small moments, and the leaning is enough. A relationship where you get it right most of the time, and repair the times you do not, is a relationship where your partner keeps their agency and you keep your sanity. That is the target, not perfection, and it is well within reach.

The through-line

Refusing to rescue does not mean refusing to help. It means changing the kind of help you give, from the sort that takes over to the sort that keeps your partner in charge of their own life. Ask before you help. Offer choices instead of verdicts. Share responsibility instead of transferring it. Let your partner make choices you would not make, and aim your help at building their capacity rather than replacing it. None of this is colder than rescue. It is warmer, because it treats your partner as a whole adult rather than a problem you are managing.

There is a moment, though, when even the most careful, choice-honoring help is not enough, and you have to do something rescue never requires: set a limit. Not a limit on your partner, but on yourself, on what you will and will not do. Boundaries are where supporting partners most often lose their nerve, because a boundary can feel like a punishment or a withdrawal of love. It is neither, when it is built correctly. The next chapter shows how to build one that protects you without attacking your partner.

Chapter 5: Boundaries That Are Not Punishment

For years, Lorien tried to control the drinking. His partner Evanthe drank more on bad nights, and the bad nights had gotten more frequent since the trauma that reshaped their lives. Lorien poured bottles down the sink. He counted cans. He delivered speeches. He extracted promises that lasted until the next hard evening. None of it worked, and all of it turned him into someone he did not like, a warden in his own home, furious and pleading by turns. He thought he was setting boundaries. He was not. He was attempting to run another adult's behavior, which cannot be done, and the failure was eating him alive.

The turning point came when a counselor asked Lorien a question that reorganized everything. "You keep telling me what you want Evanthe to stop doing. What are you going to do." Lorien had no answer, because it had never occurred to him that a boundary was about his own behavior rather than hers. That single reframe is the subject of this chapter, and it is the reframe that turns boundaries from another form of control into genuine self-protection. A real boundary is not a rule you impose on your partner. It is a decision about what you will do.

The most common mistake

Most people, when they try to set a boundary, actually issue a command. "You need to stop calling me at work." "You can't take it out on me anymore." "You have to go to therapy." These sound like boundaries and feel like boundaries, but they are attempts to control someone else's actions, and they fail for a simple reason: you do not control someone else's actions. You only control your own. When your boundary depends on your partner's compliance, you have handed them the power to violate it, and you have set yourself up for the exact battle that has been exhausting you.

The fix is to move the boundary onto your own side of the line, where you actually have authority. Instead of "you need to stop calling me at work," the owned version is, "If you call me at work when it isn't an emergency, I'm going to let it go to voicemail and call you back at lunch." Instead of "you can't take it out on me," it is, "If you start yelling, I'm going to leave the room and come back when things are calmer." Notice what changed. The boundary no longer requires your partner to do anything. It describes what you will do, which is the only thing you can actually guarantee.

The Owned Fence. A real boundary describes what you will do, not what your partner must do. You build the fence on your own land, where you have the authority to build it, and you stop trying to build it on theirs, where you never did.

Why the reframe changes everything

This is not a word game. Moving the boundary onto your own side changes the whole emotional structure of the situation. When your boundary is a command, every interaction becomes a contest of wills, and your partner's trauma often makes them more, not less, likely to resist being controlled, because control may echo the very powerlessness they are trying to recover from. You end up fighting your partner's history as well as your partner.

When your boundary is about your own behavior, there is nothing to fight. You are not telling your partner what to do. You are telling them what to expect from you, and then following through calmly. There is no ultimatum, no threat, no attempt to force. There is only a person who has decided how they will act, and who acts that way. Strangely, this is far more likely to change the situation than any command ever was, because your partner now faces real, predictable consequences that come not from your anger but from your steadiness. But even that is not the point. The point is that you are protected either way, whether or not your partner changes, because your boundary depends only on you.

Boundaries are not walls

Supporting partners often resist boundaries because they confuse them with walls, and a wall does feel like a withdrawal of love. A wall shuts the other person out. A boundary does the opposite. It makes closeness sustainable, because it lets you stay in the relationship without being consumed by it.

Think of it physically. A boundary is a fence, not a fortress. A fence marks where your land ends and your partner's begins, and a good fence makes good neighbors precisely because everyone knows where they stand. It does not mean you love your partner less or want them gone. It means you have a self, with limits, and you are letting your partner know where those limits are so that both of you can live alongside them. The partners who never set boundaries do not love more than the ones who do. They love until there is nothing left, and then they collapse or explode, which serves no one.

When Lorien stopped trying to control Evanthe's drinking and started setting owned boundaries instead, the drinking did not immediately stop. That is important, and we will come back to it. What changed first was Lorien. He stopped pouring out bottles. Instead he told Evanthe, calmly, "I love you, and I'm not going to spend the evening with you when you're drinking like this. I'll be at my brother's, and I'll be home in the morning, and I still want to be married to you." Then he went. The first time, Evanthe was enraged and frightened and accused him of abandoning her. He came home in the morning, as promised, warm and unmoved. He was not punishing her. He was declining to participate in something that was harming him, while making clear that he was not leaving the marriage. Over time, the predictability of it, the total absence of a fight to push against, changed the shape of their evenings. Not all at once. But it changed.

Rewriting the command as a boundary

The practical skill here is a kind of translation, and you can learn it. Take any demand you have been making of your partner and rewrite it as a statement about your own behavior. The formula is straightforward. "If [situation], I will [action I control]." The situation is a description, not an accusation. The action is something you can do entirely on your own, without needing your partner's cooperation.

Try this week: translate one command. Write down one thing you have been trying to make your partner do or stop doing. Now rewrite it as an owned boundary using the formula: "If this happens, I will do this." Make sure the action is completely within your control. "If dinner turns into an argument about my failings, I'll clear my plate and take a walk, and we can talk when it's calmer" is an owned boundary. "You have to stop criticizing me at dinner" is a command wearing a boundary's clothes. Do the translation on paper first, where it is easier to see the difference.

The follow-through is the whole thing

A boundary you announce but do not keep is worse than no boundary at all, because it teaches your partner that your limits are empty. This is the part that frightens people, and it is where boundaries are won or lost. Setting the boundary is easy. Following through, especially the first few times, especially when your partner is upset, is hard. It will feel, in the moment, like cruelty, and your partner may tell you it is cruelty. It is not. It is the follow-through that makes the boundary real, and a real boundary is what finally lets you stop being a warden.

Follow-through does not require harshness. In fact it works best when it is calm and warm and completely reliable. You do not have to argue for your boundary, defend it, or win the other person's agreement. You simply do what you said you would do, without drama, as many times as it takes. The calm is what makes it a boundary rather than a fight. You are not trying to hurt or teach a lesson. You are just, quietly, protecting your own land.

Try this week: plan the follow-through. For the one boundary you translated, write down exactly what you will do when the situation arises, and where you will go if you need to leave, and what you will say, in one warm sentence, so you are not composing it in the heat of the moment. Rehearse the sentence. "I love you, and I'm going to step out for a bit. I'll be back." Having the plan ready is the difference between a boundary you keep and one that dissolves the first time your partner's face falls.

When the boundary shakes you

Expect the first few boundaries to cost you something internally, even when you do them perfectly. You may feel guilty, mean, selfish, or terrified that you have damaged the relationship. Those feelings are real, and they are not evidence that you did wrong. They are the feelings of someone doing something unfamiliar and important, and they tend to be loudest right when you are on the right track. We give the next chapter entirely to this reaction, because the guilt that arrives after a fair boundary is one of the main reasons supporting partners abandon their boundaries and slide back into over-functioning.

For now, hold this. A boundary that keeps you whole is not an act of aggression against your partner. It is what allows you to keep loving them without disappearing. Evanthe's drinking was Evanthe's to change, and eventually, slowly, with her own treatment and her own choices, some of it did change. What was always Lorien's, and only ever Lorien's, was the decision about how much of his own life he would sacrifice to a problem that was not his to solve. Setting boundaries was how he took that decision back.

Firm without being rigid

A good boundary is firm, but firm is not the same as rigid, and confusing the two leads supporting partners into a harshness that damages the relationship they are trying to protect. A rigid boundary is a wall that never moves, applied identically regardless of circumstance, defended as if any flexibility were weakness. A firm boundary holds reliably and can still bend for genuine reasons, chosen consciously rather than under pressure. The difference is whether you are choosing to flex or being coerced into collapsing.

Consider the difference in practice. Lorien's boundary about not spending the evening with Evanthe when she was drinking heavily was firm. It held, night after night. But when Evanthe had a genuinely terrible day, the anniversary of the event that started all of this, and drank in obvious grief rather than in the usual pattern, Lorien chose, consciously, to stay, because this was different and he decided it was worth it. That is not a broken boundary. That is a firm boundary flexed on purpose, by the person who owns it, for a reason he could name. The test is simple: are you bending because you decided to, or because you could not withstand your partner's reaction. The first is wisdom. The second is the boundary collapsing.

There is also a quieter gift in owned boundaries that supporting partners rarely anticipate. Modeled steadily, they can actually help your partner. A person recovering from trauma is often learning, slowly, that relationships can have limits without those limits meaning abandonment, that someone can say no and still stay, that closeness and boundaries can coexist. When you hold a boundary calmly and remain warmly present afterward, you demonstrate exactly that, over and over, in a way no explanation could. You are not only protecting yourself. You are showing your partner a kind of relationship they may never have seen: one where both people have edges, and the love survives the edges intact.

None of this means boundaries become easy or that your partner will thank you for them, at least not soon. It means that the goal is a boundary that is dependable enough to protect you and human enough to belong in a real relationship. Firm, warm, and occasionally, consciously, flexible. That combination is harder than either rigid rule-keeping or spineless collapse, and it is the one that actually holds a marriage together while keeping you whole inside it.

If setting boundaries is new to you, start with a small one. Do not begin with the hardest, most charged limit in your relationship, the one wrapped in years of history and fear. Begin with something modest, where the stakes are low and the follow-through is easy, so you can feel what an owned boundary is like in your body before you attempt the big ones. Confidence with boundaries is built the way confidence with anything is built, by succeeding at small versions first. A single small boundary, set clearly and kept calmly, teaches you more than any amount of reading, and it gives you a foundation of proof that you can hold a limit and the relationship survives.

Notice, too, that owned boundaries change how you feel about your partner, not only how you behave. When you were trying to control Evanthe's drinking or Sevrin's calls or anyone's anything, you lived in a state of low, constant frustration, because you were forever failing at an impossible task. When the boundary moves onto your own land, that particular frustration drains away, because you are no longer trying to do something that cannot be done. You stop being angry at your partner for not complying, because compliance was never the point. This is one of the quieter gifts of owned boundaries. They do not only protect your time and energy. They return you to a warmer feeling toward the person you are setting them with, which is, in the end, the whole reason you wanted to protect your time and energy in the first place.

The through-line

Boundaries fail when they are commands and succeed when they are decisions about your own behavior. Build the fence on your own land. Rewrite every demand as a statement of what you will do. Follow through calmly, warmly, and reliably, and expect it to shake you at first. A boundary is not a punishment or a wall. It is the thing that lets closeness continue, because it keeps you from being consumed by the very relationship you are trying to protect.

But knowing all this does not make the aftermath easy. The moment you hold a boundary, a wave often arrives, and its name is guilt. It can be strong enough to undo everything you just built. In the next chapter we face that wave directly, because learning to stay upright in it, without either drowning in it or hardening against it, is what makes every boundary in this book possible to keep.

Chapter 6: When Guilt Arrives After "No"

Maevren said no on a Thursday. Her partner Valenor had asked her to skip her sister's birthday, again, because he did not feel up to being alone that evening and did not want her out of the house. Maevren had skipped a great deal already: two weddings, most of her book club, a weekend trip she had been looking forward to for a year. This time she said, gently and clearly, that she was going to her sister's, and that she would be home by ten, and that she loved him. Valenor's face closed. He did not yell. He simply went quiet and small, and that was worse than yelling, because Maevren spent the entire party feeling like a monster. She checked her phone every few minutes. She left early. She apologized in the car on the way home to a message he had not even sent. By the time she walked in the door, she had almost convinced herself that going had been a cruel and selfish act.

Nothing Maevren did that Thursday was cruel or selfish. She protected one small evening of her own life after giving up dozens. And still the guilt came, enormous and certain, insisting she had done something terrible. That gap, between what she actually did and what the guilt told her she did, is the subject of this chapter. Guilt is one of the most powerful forces pulling supporting partners back into over-functioning, and to hold any boundary, you have to learn what guilt is and, just as important, what it is not.

Guilt is a feeling, not a fact

Here is the reframe the whole chapter rests on. Guilt is a feeling. It is not a verdict. It arrives with the force of a judgment, as if some fair court has weighed your actions and found you guilty, but there is no court. There is only a feeling in your body, and feelings, however strong, are not evidence of wrongdoing. You can feel intensely guilty while doing exactly the right thing, and you can feel no guilt at all while doing real harm. The feeling and the facts are two separate things, and the skill is to stop letting the feeling stand in for the facts.

This matters because supporting partners are especially prone to guilt that has nothing to do with wrongdoing. When you have organized your life around another person's needs, any move toward your own needs can trigger guilt, simply because it is unfamiliar and because you have trained yourself to treat your own needs as the thing that gives way. The guilt is not reporting that you did wrong. It is reporting that you did something new. Those feel identical from the inside, and telling them apart is the work.

Guilt Is Not a Verdict. Guilt after a fair "no" is a feeling, not proof that you did something wrong. The intensity of the feeling tells you nothing about the rightness of the act, and learning to hold that distinction is what lets you keep the boundaries you set.

Two kinds of guilt

Not all guilt is false, and it would be a mistake to teach yourself to ignore it entirely. Some guilt is useful. It arrives when you have actually violated your own values, and it points you toward repair. If you snapped cruelly at your partner, or broke a promise that mattered, the guilt you feel is doing its job, and the right response is to make it right. Real guilt is worth listening to.

The guilt this chapter is about is different. It is the guilt that arrives when you have protected a legitimate need of your own, and it is not pointing toward any real wrong. Maevren's guilt was this second kind. She had not violated her values. She had honored one of them, the value of staying connected to her own family and her own life, after long neglecting it. Her guilt was not a signal to repair anything. It was the discomfort of doing something she had trained herself not to do.

You can tell the two apart with a simple question, and asking it is a genuine skill. When guilt hits, ask: did I actually violate one of my own values, or did I protect a legitimate need. If you violated a value, the guilt is useful, and you should repair. If you protected a legitimate need, the guilt is the false kind, and the task is not to obey it but to sit with it until it passes, without letting it drag you back across the boundary you set.

Try this week: run the guilt check. The next time guilt hits after you have said no or held a limit, pause and ask the question in plain words: did I violate a value, or did I protect a real need. Write down which one it is and why. If it is the second kind, write the sentence: "This guilt is a feeling, not a verdict, and I am going to let it pass without undoing what I did." Reading your own reasoning back to yourself weakens the guilt's claim to be a judgment.

The backlash is not a message

There is a particular version of this that supporting partners find hardest: the guilt that comes not from inside but from your partner's reaction. Valenor did not accuse Maevren of anything. He simply went small and quiet, and his distress landed on Maevren as proof that she had harmed him. When your partner responds to your boundary with hurt, withdrawal, anger, or collapse, your guilt reads that reaction as a verdict: see, you did do something wrong, look at the damage.

But your partner's distress at your boundary is not evidence that the boundary was wrong. A person who has grown used to your over-functioning will, understandably, be upset when it changes, and their upset is real, and it is not a message that you must reverse course. You can hold both truths. Your partner is genuinely hurting, and you did not do wrong. Their reaction deserves your compassion. It does not deserve your obedience. Learning to let your partner be upset about a fair boundary, without either dismissing their feelings or surrendering to them, is one of the deepest skills in this book. It is also, done with warmth, one of the kindest, because a relationship in which one person can never be disappointed is not a relationship. It is a hostage situation with good intentions.

Riding the wave

Guilt, when you do not act on it, behaves like a wave. It rises, peaks, and falls, usually faster than you expect. The reason it feels permanent is that supporting partners almost never let it crest. They rush to make it stop, by apologizing, by undoing the boundary, by over-functioning again, and the relief of that undoing teaches them, just as in the rescue loop, to do it again. If you can tolerate the guilt for the length of one wave, without acting on it, you discover something the loop never let you learn: it passes on its own, and you are still standing, and nothing terrible happened.

The way through a wave is not to fight it or argue with it, which only makes it louder. It is to notice it, name it, and let it move through you while you decline to obey it. "This is guilt. It is here because I did something unfamiliar and good, not because I did something wrong. I am going to feel it and not fix it." Then you do the next ordinary thing, wash a dish, answer an email, and let the wave fall.

Here is where a body of research becomes practical. How you treat yourself in these moments changes how badly they go. The psychologist Kristin Neff has spent two decades studying what she calls self-compassion, the practice of responding to your own suffering the way you would respond to a friend's rather than with harsh self-criticism (Neff, 2003). In caregivers specifically, higher self-compassion is linked to lower guilt and shame, less burnout, and a greater ability to keep caring without collapsing (Neff, 2023). This is not softness for its own sake. It is the difference between a supporter who can sustain their boundaries and one who is beaten back across them by their own inner voice. When the guilt wave hits, the harsh response, calling yourself selfish and cruel, feeds the wave. The steady, friend-like response, "of course this is hard, and I still did the right thing," lets it pass.

Try this week: the friend test. When guilt tells you that you are selfish for protecting your own need, ask what you would say to a close friend in the same situation. You would almost certainly not call them cruel. You would tell them their need was legitimate and their guilt was understandable but not a verdict. Say that same thing to yourself, in the same tone. It will feel awkward. Do it anyway. Speaking to yourself as you would to someone you love is a trained skill, and it is one of the strongest guards against being pushed back into over-functioning.

What Maevren learned

Maevren did not transform overnight. The Thursday of her sister's party ended with her over-apologizing to Valenor, undoing some of the good she had done, sliding halfway back across her own line. That is how it usually goes at first. But she had done the harder half, she had gone, and over the following months she went to more things, and each time the guilt was a little less able to convince her she was a monster. Valenor, for his part, did not fall apart when she left the house, which he had feared and she had feared. He was uncomfortable, and he survived it, and his surviving it was its own quiet lesson for both of them. Some evenings he even encouraged her to go, which neither of them would have predicted.

None of this meant Maevren stopped caring about Valenor's feelings. She cared as much as ever. What changed was that his feelings stopped functioning as an automatic override on her own life. She could hold his distress and her boundary in the same two hands, and that two-handed capacity, more than any single boundary, was what let her stay both loving and present.

The apology reflex

Guilt has a favorite behavior, and it is apology. Watch a supporting partner in the grip of false guilt and you will see it: they apologize constantly, reflexively, for things that require no apology. Sorry for being tired. Sorry for wanting an evening out. Sorry for having a need. Sorry for saying no. The apology is how guilt discharges itself, and every reflexive apology quietly confirms the false verdict, teaching both people that you did something wrong when you did not.

The problem with the apology reflex is that it undoes your boundaries even when you keep them. Maevren went to her sister's party, which was the boundary, and then apologized for it in the car, over and over, which handed back most of what the boundary had won. She kept the action and surrendered the meaning. Her partner learned that going was allowed but shameful, which is barely better than not going at all. The apology said: this thing I did, that I had every right to do, was a wrong against you. That is a lie, and repeated often enough, both people come to believe it.

Breaking the reflex starts with noticing it, because it is so automatic that most people do not hear themselves doing it. Once you can hear it, you can experiment with a substitution. Where you would have apologized for a legitimate need, try replacing "I'm sorry" with a simple, non-apologetic statement of the fact, or with a thank-you where thanks fit better than sorry. "Sorry I was out so late" becomes "Thanks for holding down the evening." "Sorry I need some time to myself" becomes "I'm going to take an hour this afternoon." The information is the same. What disappears is the false confession of wrongdoing.

Try this week: swap the apology. For one week, listen for the reflexive apologies that follow your legitimate needs and boundaries. Each time you catch one, try to swap it for a plain statement or a thank-you instead. You are not becoming rude or ungrateful. You are declining to confess to a crime you did not commit. Notice how it feels to state a need without apologizing for it. For most supporting partners, it feels wrong at first and then, gradually, like standing up straight after a long time hunched.

It is worth saying plainly that the guilt does get quieter over time, though not because you talk yourself out of it in any single moment. It gets quieter because you keep acting well in spite of it, and your nervous system slowly learns that these fair boundaries do not, in fact, lead to catastrophe. The first time you hold a limit through a wave of guilt, it is agony. The tenth time, it is merely uncomfortable. The fiftieth time, the guilt may barely register, because you have accumulated a long record of evidence that protecting a legitimate need is safe and right. You are not trying to feel no guilt. You are trying to stop letting guilt make your decisions, and that shift, repeated, is what eventually quiets the feeling itself.

Remember that none of this requires you to become hard. The goal is not to feel less, to care less about your partner's disappointment, or to build a shell that nothing gets through. The goal is to feel the guilt fully and still act well, to let your partner's hurt matter to you and still hold your ground. That combination, soft heart and steady spine, is harder than either coldness or collapse, and it is the one that keeps you both human. You can be tender and firm at the same time. In fact, in this relationship, you will have to be.

The through-line

Guilt is a feeling, not a verdict, and the guilt that follows a fair boundary is almost always the false kind, reporting only that you did something unfamiliar. You can tell it apart from useful guilt by asking whether you violated a value or protected a real need. You can survive your partner's distress without treating it as proof of wrongdoing. And you can ride the guilt wave to its natural fall, especially when you respond to yourself with the steadiness you would offer a friend rather than with self-attack. These are the skills that keep the boundaries of the last chapter from dissolving the first time your partner's face falls.

So far this book has worked mostly on your own side of the relationship, your load, your roles, your rescues, your limits, your guilt. It is time to turn toward your partner's actual recovery, and toward one of the most delicate conversations a supporting partner ever has: how to talk about professional help. Many supporting partners either avoid the subject entirely or push so hard that it backfires. In the next chapter we find the narrow path between, the way to open the door to treatment without appointing yourself the treatment.

Chapter 7: Talking About Treatment Without Becoming Treatment

Noélin had a folder. Inside it were printouts about three trauma therapists, a summary of a treatment approach she had researched, a list of reasons Alaris should get professional help, and a rebuttal for every objection she expected him to raise. She had been building the folder for months, and she planned to present it to Alaris over dinner, the way you might present a legal case. She was certain that if she could just lay out the evidence clearly enough, he would finally agree to go. Alaris, fifty-three, had lived with untreated post-traumatic stress for most of their marriage, and Noélin, fifty, was out of patience and out of ideas. The folder was her last, best argument.

The folder never worked, and it was never going to, and understanding why is the key to this entire chapter. When you argue for change, the person you are arguing with tends to argue back, defending the very position you are trying to move them off of. The harder Noélin pushed for therapy, the more Alaris would explain why therapy was pointless, and each explanation would leave him more committed to not going. She was not opening the door to treatment. She was, without meaning to, helping Alaris talk himself out of it. There is a better way, and it comes from the people who have studied how humans actually change their minds.

The righting reflex strikes again

We met the righting reflex two chapters ago, the urge to fix a struggling person by supplying the obvious solution (Miller & Rollnick, 2013). Nowhere is it stronger than around the subject of professional help. You can see so clearly that your partner needs treatment. You have the printouts. You have the arguments. And so you deliver them, again and again, and you cannot understand why it does not work, because from where you stand the answer is so obvious.

Here is the mechanism. When you make the case for change, you take up all the pro-change arguments, which leaves your partner holding all the against-change arguments. In the strange arithmetic of persuasion, people believe what they hear themselves say. So the more you argue for therapy, the more your partner voices reasons against it, and the more they hear themselves reject it, the more entrenched they become. The clinicians who developed a method for exactly these conversations found that arguing for change reliably produces the opposite of change (Miller & Rollnick, 2013). Your certainty, delivered as pressure, becomes the thing your partner pushes against.

Offer, Don't Operate. You can open the door to treatment. You cannot walk through it for your partner. Your job is to make the door visible and easy to reach, and then to stop pushing, because the pushing is what holds it shut.

Let them make the case

The counterintuitive move, and the heart of the method, is to stop making the argument for change and instead help your partner explore their own reasons. Most people who resist treatment are not simply opposed. They are ambivalent. Part of them wants relief and part of them is afraid, and when you argue only for the wanting-relief side, they get stuck defending the afraid side. If you can instead invite them to voice their own mixed feelings, including their own reasons for wanting things to be different, they begin to hear themselves make the case, and that is the only case that ever moves anyone.

This is quieter and slower than presenting a folder. It sounds like curiosity rather than advocacy. "How do you feel about how things have been going." "Is there any part of you that wishes it were different." "What would have to be true for you to consider talking to someone." These are not trick questions designed to lead your partner to your conclusion. They are genuine invitations to explore, and they only work if you can tolerate whatever answer comes, including "no part of me wants that right now." When your partner does voice a reason for change, however small, your job is not to pounce on it and build your case. It is to be curious about it. "Tell me more about that." The reasons your partner speaks out loud are worth a thousand of yours.

The invitation, not the ultimatum

There is a place for stating clearly that you hope your partner will get help, and for offering to make it easy. The difference between an invitation and an ultimatum is not the content but the pressure behind it, and your partner can feel the difference instantly. An invitation is offered once, warmly, and then left open. An ultimatum is repeated, escalated, and attached to consequences meant to force compliance.

An invitation sounds like this. "I love you, and I've watched how hard this has been. I think talking to a professional could help, and I'd support you completely if you decided to, I'd help you find someone, come with you, whatever you needed. And it's your call, and I'm not going to keep bringing it up." Then, crucially, you do not keep bringing it up. You said it clearly once. Nagging does not add information; it only adds pressure, and pressure holds the door shut. The hardest part of the invitation is the silence after it, the discipline of not returning to the subject every week. That silence is not giving up. It is respect, and respect is often what finally lets a person move.

Try this week: draft your one invitation. Write out, in your own words, a single warm invitation for your partner to consider professional help. Include three things: that you love them, that you think help could ease things, and that the decision is entirely theirs and you will support whatever they choose. Then add the sentence you will actually have to keep: "I'm not going to keep pushing this." Read it over and cut anything that sounds like an argument or a threat. You are opening a door, not winning a case.

When to stop bringing it up

Supporting partners often ask how many times they should raise the subject of treatment. For most situations, the answer is close to once, clearly, and then as an open standing offer they do not repeat. This feels wrong, because it feels like doing nothing while your partner suffers. But repeatedly raising it does not move your partner closer to help. It moves them further away, and it turns you into the nagging spouse, which corrodes the intimacy that might otherwise draw your partner toward change.

There is a specific trap worth naming. Some supporting partners, in their eagerness to help, actually accommodate their partner around treatment in ways that undermine it, and some inadvertently support avoidance of care. Partners have been known to collude in a survivor's avoidance, even encouraging them to skip or drop out of therapy when it stirs up hard feelings, because seeing their partner distressed after a session is painful (Fredman et al., 2014). If your partner is in treatment, one of the most useful things you can do is not to undermine it when it gets hard, and hard is often a sign it is working rather than a sign to quit. Encouraging therapy is support. Sitting in on it, second-guessing it, or trying to do a home version of it is operating, and operating is not yours to do.

The offer you can always make

Even when your partner is not ready for their own treatment, there is one form of professional help entirely within your control, and supporting partners routinely overlook it. You can get help for yourself. You do not need your partner's permission or participation to talk to a therapist about your own exhaustion, your own guilt, your own life inside this relationship. This is not a consolation prize or a way of secretly pressuring your partner. It is a legitimate good in itself, and it sometimes shifts the whole system, because a supporting partner who is steadier and less depleted changes what is possible between the two of you.

There is even a form of couple-based therapy designed for exactly these situations, developed specifically to work with trauma inside the relationship rather than around it (Monson & Fredman, 2012), in which both partners work together with a professional on how trauma is affecting the bond. A small trial of one such present-focused approach found meaningful reductions in PTSD symptoms across treatment (Pukay-Martin et al., 2015). Whether or not that fits your situation, the broader point stands. Getting help is not something you can only do once your partner agrees to it. You can start on your own side, today, and doing so is one of the clearest ways to model that reaching for help is a strength rather than a surrender.

What actually happened with Alaris

Noélin never presented the folder. Instead, over several months, she stopped arguing and started asking, and she made her single warm invitation and then, with great difficulty, went quiet on the subject. She also, for the first time, found a therapist for herself, to deal with her own years of depletion. Nothing happened quickly. Alaris did not have a sudden change of heart. But one evening, unprompted, he asked her how her sessions were going, and a few weeks after that he asked, almost casually, whether she thought the person she was seeing might know someone he could talk to. He went, eventually, on his own timeline, for his own reasons, which he could name because he had been allowed to find them himself rather than having Noélin's reasons pressed on him.

It is worth acknowledging that this does not always happen. Some partners never seek treatment, and no amount of skillful invitation can guarantee otherwise, because the choice is genuinely theirs. If that is your situation, the chapters on boundaries and on supporting yourself matter even more, because they are about the parts of the picture you can control regardless of what your partner decides. What you can offer is a visible, reachable door and a relationship worth walking toward. What you cannot do is walk through the door for them, and the sooner you stop trying, the more likely they are to walk through it themselves.

Reading the moment

Even a perfect invitation lands badly at the wrong moment, and timing is a skill worth developing. The worst time to raise professional help is in the middle of a crisis or a fight, when your partner is flooded and defensive and any suggestion sounds like an attack or an accusation that they are the problem. Yet the middle of a crisis is exactly when the subject feels most urgent to you, which is why so many of these conversations happen at precisely the wrong time and go precisely as badly as they can.

Better moments tend to be calm ones, when connection is good and no one is under threat. A quiet evening, a walk, an ordinary afternoon. The conversation goes better when your partner feels close to you and safe with you, because then the suggestion of help arrives inside a relationship rather than inside a conflict. This requires patience, holding the subject until a decent moment arrives instead of blurting it out the instant the impulse strikes. Waiting for the right moment is not the same as avoiding the subject. It is choosing the conditions under which your words have a chance of being heard.

There is also the situation where your partner says yes and then stalls, agrees to get help and never books the appointment, or books it and cancels. This is common, and it is not necessarily a lie or a dodge. Ambivalence does not vanish because someone said yes once; the frightened part reasserts itself the moment the appointment becomes real. The temptation here is to take over, to book it yourself, to drive them there against a fresh wave of reluctance, which drops you straight back into rescuing and operating. The steadier response is to keep the door open and the choice theirs. "I noticed the appointment didn't happen. No pressure. The offer to help you set it up still stands whenever you want it." Then you wait again, which is hard, and which respects that the walking-through is theirs to do.

Noélin had to sit through several of these stalls with Alaris, each one testing her resolve not to grab the wheel. He agreed, then delayed, then agreed again. She held the door open without pushing through it, and eventually he walked through on his own, which meant that when the work got hard, as it did, it was his work, chosen by him, and he stayed with it in a way he never would have stayed with something she had forced.

Underneath all the technique in this chapter is a single change of posture, and it is worth naming on its own. You are moving from trying to produce an outcome in your partner to trying to create the conditions in which they can choose. That is a genuine surrender, and it is uncomfortable, because it means letting go of the illusion that if you just find the right words, the right argument, the right folder, you can make your partner get help. You cannot make them. You never could. What you can do is love them, keep the door visible, and get help for yourself, and it turns out that this posture, humble as it feels, moves people more often than all the pushing ever did.

And if your partner never chooses treatment, that outcome, painful as it is, does not mean you failed at this chapter. You are responsible for offering the door, not for the choice made in front of it. Some people, for reasons of their own, are not ready, or not willing, or not able, within the timeframe you are living in. Holding that reality without either abandoning your partner or destroying yourself trying to force them is its own hard and honorable work. You keep the door open, you keep your own life intact, and you let the choice remain where it has always been, which is with them.

The through-line

Arguing for treatment produces resistance, because people believe what they hear themselves say, and pushing leaves your partner voicing all the reasons against. The way through is to stop advocating and start inviting: to help your partner explore their own ambivalence, to offer a single warm invitation and then respect the silence after it, and to support treatment without undermining it or trying to deliver it yourself. And there is one form of help you never have to wait for, which is help for you. You open the door. You do not operate the patient.

There is a risk in a book like this one, and it is time to correct for it. We have spent seven chapters on managing trauma's effect on your relationship, which can make it sound as if your relationship is nothing but a trauma to be managed. It is not, or it does not have to be. Underneath the symptom management is a relationship, with affection and friendship and laughter and desire and shared dreams, and that relationship has often gone quiet under the weight of everything else. The next chapter is about turning back toward it, about keeping love reciprocal rather than letting it collapse into an endless caregiving arrangement.

Chapter 8: Keeping Love Reciprocal

Solenne was asked a question by a friend that she could not answer. They were having coffee, and the friend, who knew about Auren, said, "That's a lot you carry. What does Auren do for you these days." Solenne opened her mouth and found nothing there. She could list, without pausing, everything she did for Auren. She could not, in that moment, name a single thing he did for her. Not because he did nothing, she realized later, but because she had stopped noticing, and, worse, had stopped letting him. Somewhere in the years of managing his trauma, their marriage had quietly become a one-way street, and Solenne had been so busy giving that she had forgotten a relationship is supposed to run in both directions.

That silence at the coffee shop is where this chapter begins. A relationship touched by trauma tends to narrow. Bit by bit, everything becomes about the trauma, about symptoms, appointments, triggers, and coping, until the trauma is the only room left in the house. The affection, the friendship, the laughter, the desire, the shared dreams, all the things that made this a love rather than a care arrangement, get pushed into a corner and gather dust. This chapter is about turning back toward them, because a love that has become nothing but caregiving is a love in danger, no matter how devoted the caregiver.

The ledger that runs one way

Healthy relationships keep a rough, unspoken balance of giving and receiving. Not a strict tally, and not a transaction, but a general sense that both people give and both people receive, over time, in their own currencies. When trauma enters, this balance often collapses. The supporting partner gives more and more, and the partner with trauma, absorbed in survival, gives less and less, and everyone accepts this as the necessary shape of things. For a season, it may be. Held for years, it becomes corrosive, because human beings are not built to give endlessly while receiving nothing, and a person who only gives eventually runs dry and, often, grows quietly resentful without knowing why.

The fix is not to demand that your struggling partner suddenly match your output. It is to reopen the flow in both directions, which starts with a change in you: you have to be willing to receive again. Many supporting partners, without realizing it, have stopped letting their partner give to them. They have decided their partner is too fragile, too burdened, too unwell to be leaned on for anything, and so they refuse all offers and ask for nothing. This looks like consideration. It is also, unintentionally, a way of keeping the relationship one-directional and keeping your partner in the role of patient rather than partner.

The Two-Way Ledger. Love stays alive when both giving and receiving keep moving. A relationship that runs in one direction is not more loving for it. It is slowly starving, and the cure is not to give more but to let yourself receive again.

Letting your partner give

Here is a truth that surprises supporting partners. Letting your partner do things for you is not a burden you place on them. It is often a gift you give them. People with trauma histories frequently feel useless, like a weight their partner has to carry, and that sense of being nothing but a problem is corrosive to recovery. When you let your partner contribute, cook a meal, comfort you on your hard day, handle a task, offer real support, you give them the experience of being capable and valuable rather than only needy. That experience of competence is one of the basic human needs, and meeting it lifts people rather than draining them (Deci & Ryan, 2000).

Consider Sorell, thirty-three, and their partner Virel, who has post-traumatic stress after surviving a disaster that killed people she loved. For two years Sorell protected Virel from everything, including from Sorell's own bad days, presenting a constant untroubled front so as not to add to Virel's load. Virel, it turned out, hated this. She told Sorell, in a rare sharp moment, "You won't let me be your partner. You only let me be your project." It stung because it was true. When Sorell began, cautiously, to let Virel in, to admit when work was hard, to accept comfort, to let Virel take care of them when they were sick, something shifted for both of them. Virel got to be a person who gives rather than only a person who is managed. Sorell got a partner back. It did not fix Virel's trauma. It did remind them both that they were still, underneath everything, two people who loved each other rather than a caregiver and a case.

Making room for the non-trauma relationship

Beyond the balance of giving and receiving, there is the simple matter of what you actually do together, and in trauma-narrowed relationships the plain answer is often: manage the trauma, and little else. You have to deliberately rebuild the parts of the relationship that have nothing to do with the condition, because they will not return on their own.

This means protecting time and activities that are not about trauma at all. A walk where the rule is that neither of you raises the hard subject. A show you watch together for no reason but enjoyment. A meal out, if that is possible, or a meal in that you make an occasion of. An inside joke revived. A shared plan for something in the future, however small, a garden, a trip, a project, because couples who have stopped imagining a future together have lost something that dreams, even modest ones, restore. None of this denies the trauma. It simply refuses to let the trauma be the only thing. Your partner is not their diagnosis, and neither is your marriage, and the way you keep that true is by regularly living the parts of your life that the trauma does not touch.

Try this week: reintroduce one ordinary thing. Choose one activity you used to share that had nothing to do with trauma, and bring it back, in whatever reduced form is realistic. It does not have to be ambitious. Fifteen minutes of a card game, a short walk, cooking one meal together. The only rule is that it is for pleasure and connection, not for processing or coping. If your partner cannot manage it this week, that is information, not failure, and you can try a smaller version. The point is to reopen a room in the house that has been shut.

Affection and desire

Affection often goes quiet in trauma-affected relationships, and physical intimacy, in particular, can become complicated, sometimes because of the trauma itself, sometimes because the relationship has drifted into a parent-child or nurse-patient shape that has little room for desire. This is delicate territory, and it does not resolve on command. But it is worth naming, because supporting partners often suffer the loss of this part of the relationship in silence, assuming it is selfish to want it or hopeless to raise it.

It is neither selfish nor hopeless, though it does require care. The path back to physical closeness, when trauma is involved, runs through safety, patience, and consent rather than through pressure or scheduling. Small, non-demanding affection, a hand held, sitting close, a hug that asks for nothing, often has to come back before anything more does, and it may need to be rebuilt slowly and with explicit conversation about what feels safe. If sexual difficulties are rooted in the trauma itself, this is an area where professional help, for your partner or for both of you, can matter, and it is not a failure to seek it. What you can do on your own is refuse to let the affectionate, desiring part of your relationship be quietly written off, and keep the door to it open with patience rather than pressure.

The audit you have been avoiding

Most supporting partners can recite what they give. Far fewer have looked squarely at what they receive, partly because they suspect the answer will be painful, and partly because they have trained themselves to believe their own needs do not count. Looking anyway is important, not to build a case against your partner, but to see the actual shape of the relationship clearly, so you can decide what to reopen.

Try this week: the reciprocity audit. On paper, make two columns. In the first, list what you give your partner in a typical week. In the second, list what you receive from them. Do not perform either list; be candid. If the second column is short, resist two temptations: the temptation to blame your partner, and the temptation to pretend it does not matter. Instead, pick one specific thing you could begin to receive again, comfort on a hard day, help with one task, a genuine conversation about your life, and this week, let your partner give it to you. Letting yourself be given to is the exercise. It is harder than it sounds, and it is the beginning of a two-way relationship.

When it stays lopsided

It is only fair to say that some relationships remain lopsided, at least for long stretches, and that reciprocity is not always available in the measure you need. A partner in an acute phase of trauma may genuinely have little to give for a time, and expecting otherwise is neither kind nor realistic. The aim of this chapter is not a perfect fifty-fifty ledger, which no relationship achieves anyway. It is to interrupt the drift toward a relationship that runs entirely one way, to keep receiving where you can, to let your partner contribute where they are able, and to protect the non-trauma parts of your bond so they do not vanish.

And if you find, over a long period, that the relationship gives you almost nothing, no affection, no support, no companionship, no reciprocity of any kind, that is important information about your own wellbeing and your own choices, information the next two chapters will help you use. For now, the work is to stop assuming the one-way street is simply how it must be, and to reopen the flow, in both directions, wherever it can be reopened.

Solenne went home from that coffee shop and, over the following weeks, started letting Auren back in. She told him about her own hard days instead of hiding them. She let him make dinner when he offered, even though she could have done it faster. She asked him, one evening, to just hold her, with no agenda, and he did, and she cried, and he was, for once, the one offering comfort rather than receiving it. It was a small thing. It was also the first genuinely two-way moment their marriage had held in a long time, and it reminded them both that it was still, underneath all the management, a marriage.

Friendship is the ground floor

Underneath the affection and the desire and the shared dreams, there is something more basic that trauma tends to erode first and that most supporting partners forget to rebuild: friendship. The plain enjoyment of each other's company. The ability to talk about nothing, laugh at something dumb, be easy together. When a relationship narrows to symptom management, the friendship is usually the first casualty, because friendship needs unstructured time and lightness, and both of those vanish under the weight of caregiving. You can still love someone you are no longer friends with, but it is a heavier, lonelier love, and it is worth noticing when it has happened.

Rebuilding the friendship does not require anything dramatic. It requires small, repeated moments of being companionable rather than clinical. Telling your partner something that happened at work, not because it needs solving but because that is what friends do. Sharing an article, a song, a bit of gossip. Asking your partner's opinion about something ordinary and unrelated to their condition, which reminds them, and you, that they have opinions about ordinary things, that they are a whole person with a mind and a sense of humor and preferences about the world. These moments are easy to skip when everything feels serious, and skipping them is how the friendship quietly dies.

Sorell realized, at one point, that they had not asked Virel a light, curious, friend-type question in months. Every question had been a check-in: how are you feeling, did you sleep, was today hard. Useful questions, all of them, and also a kind of surveillance that had crowded out the ordinary curiosity friends have about each other. When Sorell started asking Virel what she thought about things again, a film, a piece of news, a plan a mutual friend had, Virel visibly brightened. She was being treated as a person with a perspective rather than a patient with a status to report.

The friendship, it turned out, had not died. It had only been buried under check-ins, and it came back the moment it was watered.

This is the ground floor of a two-way relationship, and it is the easiest to rebuild because it costs so little. You do not need energy you do not have or time you cannot find. You only need to remember, in the small moments, to be your partner's friend and not only their caretaker, to bring lightness and curiosity into a house that has grown too heavy. The affection and the rest tend to follow, but they follow the friendship, and the friendship follows a single decision: to enjoy this person again, on purpose, starting now.

A final encouragement, because this chapter asks for something that can feel frivolous when life is hard: permission to enjoy your relationship again. In the middle of managing trauma, joy can seem like a luxury you have not earned, or a betrayal of how serious things are. It is neither. The affection, the friendship, the laughter, the shared life, these are not distractions from the real work. For most couples, they are the real work, the thing the whole relationship exists to protect. Turning back toward them is not turning away from your partner's recovery. It is remembering what the recovery is for.

The through-line

A relationship touched by trauma narrows toward symptom management and drifts into a one-way street, and the cure is not to give more but to reopen the flow in both directions. Let your partner give to you, which meets their need to be capable rather than only needy. Rebuild the parts of the relationship that have nothing to do with trauma. Keep affection and desire from being quietly written off. And take clear stock of what you receive, so you can begin to receive it again. Love stays alive on a two-way ledger, not a one-way sacrifice.

All of this reopening asks something of you, and it is something many supporting partners have long since run out of: energy, steadiness, a self with reserves. You cannot pour from an empty cup, and by now yours may be close to empty. The next chapter turns fully toward you, toward building the real, structured support that a supporting partner needs and almost never has, because your maintenance is not a luxury or a distraction from the relationship. It is part of what keeps the relationship alive.

Chapter 9: The Supporting Partner Needs Support Too

Caelan realized he had no one to call. It happened on a bad night, after Auren-like hours of managing his partner's crisis, when the worst had finally passed and Caelan sat alone in the kitchen at two in the morning, shaking a little, needing to talk to a human being who was on his side. He scrolled through his phone. His closest friend had drifted away during the two years Caelan had spent canceling plans. His brother did not know the half of it. He had no therapist. His hobbies had ended so long ago he could barely remember them. He had built his entire life around supporting his partner and, in doing so, had dismantled every source of support for himself. He was, he saw with a cold clarity, completely alone in the middle of a job that no one should do alone.

Caelan's two-in-the-morning kitchen is where a great many supporting partners eventually find themselves, and it is the direct result of a belief this chapter exists to dismantle: the belief that the supporter does not need support. You do. Not as a luxury, not as a reward for good behavior, not as a distraction from the real work of caring for your partner, but as a basic requirement of being able to care at all. This chapter is about building the support that supporting partners almost never have, and about why doing so is one of the most responsible things you can do for the relationship, not a betrayal of it.

The cost you have been absorbing

There is a name for what trauma does to the people around the survivor, and naming it matters, because supporting partners so often believe their exhaustion is a personal failing rather than a known phenomenon. Researchers describe how a survivor's trauma affects not only them but their partner, so that the partner develops their own distress, their own symptoms of stress, their own version of the wound, absorbed through years of closeness and caring (Nelson Goff & Smith, 2005). The model these researchers built treats the couple as a single system in which trauma moves between people, which means your struggle is not separate from your partner's and not a sign of weakness. It is what happens to a person who stands close to trauma for a long time.

This has a practical consequence. If your distress is real and predictable rather than imaginary and shameful, then it deserves real support rather than private endurance. You would not tell someone carrying a heavy physical load for years that they should feel nothing and need nothing. The load you carry is invisible, which is exactly why you and everyone around you keep forgetting it is there. It is there. And a load that heavy requires more than one person's shoulders.

Oxygen First. A supporter running on empty cannot support anyone. Your own maintenance is not stolen from the relationship. It is part of the relationship's maintenance, and neglecting it does not make you more devoted. It makes you less able to do the thing you are neglecting yourself for.

Why supporters isolate

The isolation Caelan discovered does not happen by accident, and understanding how it happens helps you reverse it. Supporting partners isolate through a thousand small, reasonable-seeming choices. You cancel plans because tonight is a bad night, and then you stop making plans because so many nights are bad. You do not tell friends the truth because it feels disloyal to your partner, or too heavy to lay on anyone, so your friendships grow thin and eventually vanish for lack of anything real passing through them. You drop your hobbies because there is no time and no energy, and because it feels selfish to spend an hour on yourself when your partner is suffering. Each choice makes sense. Together they wall you into a room with only your partner's trauma for company.

There is also a subtler driver: privacy that curdles into secrecy. Many supporting partners feel they must protect their partner's story, which is a decent instinct, and they extend it into never speaking to anyone about their own experience, which is a harmful mistake. You can protect your partner's privacy and still get support for yourself. The two are not in conflict. You are allowed to tell a trusted friend or a therapist that your life is hard right now, without betraying your partner's confidence, and doing so is not disloyalty. It is survival.

The three kinds of support you need

A support plan for a supporting partner has three parts, and most supporting partners have let all three collapse. The first is people: friends and family who know at least some of what you carry and who are on your side. Not people you must manage or perform for, but people with whom you can be the one who needs something. The second is professional support: your own therapist or counselor, or a support group for partners and family members of trauma survivors, where your experience is understood and you are not the strong one holding everything together. The third is a self, the interests, rest, and private space that make you a person rather than a function. All three matter, and all three can be rebuilt, though it takes deliberate effort, because none of them will return on their own.

Consider Avenor, whose partner has complex trauma, and who spent three years as a full-time, unsupported supporter before she nearly broke. Her recovery did not begin with a grand gesture. It began with one phone call to one old friend, in which she said, for the first time out loud, "I'm really struggling, and I haven't told anyone." That single conversation cracked the isolation open. Over the following months she added a support group for partners of trauma survivors, then, eventually, a therapist of her own, then, slowly, one reclaimed evening a week that was hers alone. None of it fixed her partner. All of it made her able to keep going without disappearing, and it made her, by her partner's own account, easier to be around, because she was no longer running on fumes and resentment.

Try this week: map your people. Write down the names of anyone who could be a source of support for you, even a thin or lapsed connection. Then pick one, just one, and reach out this week with something real, not "how are you" but "I've been having a hard time and I miss you." You are not asking them to fix anything. You are cracking the isolation open, the way Avenor did, with one true sentence to one person.

Rest and private space are not indulgences

Supporting partners are often chronically short on two things that sound like luxuries and are actually necessities: rest and private space. Rest, because vigilance is exhausting and a mind that is always half on someone else never fully recovers. Private space, because a person with no room of their own, literal or figurative, slowly loses the sense of being a separate self, which is precisely the erosion this whole book is trying to reverse.

Private space does not require a spare room or a weekend away, though those help if you can get them. It can be a walk you take alone, a bath with the door closed, an hour at a cafe, a standing arrangement where a friend or family member is with your partner so you can be somewhere else being yourself. The point is that you regularly go somewhere, physically or mentally, that is yours, where you are not monitoring, not managing, not on duty. This is not abandonment. Everyone, including your partner, is better served by a supporter who has a self to return to.

Try this week: claim one hour. Schedule one hour this week that is entirely yours, protected in advance, spent on something that is for you and not for your partner or the relationship. Put it in the calendar. Arrange whatever needs arranging so you can actually take it. Then take it, and notice the guilt if it comes, and let it pass, because by now you know that guilt is a feeling and not a verdict. One protected hour is small. It is also a declaration that you still exist.

Getting your own professional support

The single most useful step many supporting partners can take is to get a therapist of their own, and it is worth saying plainly because so many supporters assume therapy is only for the person with the diagnosis. It is not. Your own counseling is a place to put down the load for an hour, to be the one who is cared for, to sort out your guilt and your boundaries and your grief with someone trained to help. It also models something important for your partner: that reaching for professional help is normal and strengthening rather than shameful.

Research on caregivers points in the same direction. Higher self-compassion and adequate support are linked to lower burnout and a greater ability to keep caring over time (Neff, 2023). You cannot self-compassion your way out of a structural lack of support, and this chapter is not asking you to. It is asking you to build the actual scaffolding, people, professional help, rest, and a self, that makes it possible to keep loving your partner without being consumed. If cost or access is a barrier to professional help, support groups for partners and family members of trauma survivors, many of them low cost or free, are a genuine resource, and finding one for your situation is a concrete step worth taking.

Try this week: take one professional step. Take a single concrete action toward professional support for yourself. Look up therapists who take your insurance. Find one support group for partners of trauma survivors and note when it meets. Send one email or make one call. You do not have to complete the whole journey this week. You only have to take the first real step, because the first step is the one supporting partners keep putting off forever.

Waiting for permission that never comes

Many supporting partners have a specific, unspoken belief that keeps them from taking any of the steps in this chapter: the belief that they need permission to rest, and that the permission has to come from outside, from their partner, from circumstances easing, from some future moment when things are finally calm enough. So they wait. They will get support once the crisis passes. They will see a friend once their partner is doing better. They will reclaim a hobby once there is time. The permission never arrives, because the crisis does not fully pass and there is never enough time, and the waiting becomes a life.

No one is coming to give you permission. That is the hard and freeing truth of this chapter. Your partner, absorbed in their own survival, is unlikely to notice that you are drowning and hand you a life vest. Circumstances will not conveniently calm down and grant you a season of rest. The permission has to be one you give yourself, on the grounds established throughout this book: that you are a person with legitimate needs, that your maintenance is part of the relationship's maintenance, and that a depleted supporter serves no one. You do not have to earn rest by suffering enough first. You are allowed to rest because you are a human being with limits, which you have been all along.

Giving yourself permission is one thing; making it logistically possible is another, and the logistics are worth planning rather than leaving to chance. If taking an hour or an evening for yourself means someone needs to be with your partner, or means arranging your day around it, then arrange it in advance rather than hoping a gap appears. A friend or family member who can spend time with your partner. A standing evening that is yours. A regular arrangement rather than a rare, guilt-soaked exception. Respite that depends on everything lining up perfectly will never happen. Respite that is planned, scheduled, and defended in advance, like any other important appointment, actually happens.

Caelan, after his two-in-the-morning night, did not wait for permission. He gave it to himself, and then he handled the logistics, arranging for his brother to spend Wednesday evenings with his partner so that Caelan could go to a support group and, afterward, simply sit in a cafe being a person for an hour. It was not selfish and it did not weaken his care. It was the scaffolding that let his care continue, built by the only person who was ever going to build it, which was Caelan himself.

If everything in this chapter feels impossible right now, if you have no energy for phone calls or hobbies or private hours, start with the smallest possible version and let that be enough for now. One text to one person.

One search for one support group. One protected fifteen minutes. You are not required to rebuild your entire support system this week, and trying to do it all at once is its own way of setting yourself up to do nothing. The isolation was built one small choice at a time, and it comes apart the same way, one small choice at a time. Pick one. That is the whole assignment.

There is a version of self-neglect that disguises itself as virtue, and it is worth catching. Running yourself into the ground for your partner can feel noble, even loving, and supporting partners sometimes wear their depletion like proof of devotion. It is not proof of anything except that you are heading toward collapse. The most loving thing a depleted supporter can do is refuse to be a martyr, because a martyr, in the end, is no use to the person they were martyring themselves for. Choosing to stay whole is not the opposite of loving your partner. It is a condition of being able to keep doing it.

The through-line

The supporter needs support, not as a reward or an indulgence but as a basic requirement of being able to support at all. Your distress is real and predictable, the known cost of standing close to trauma, and it deserves genuine support rather than private endurance. Rebuild the three things isolation took: your people, your professional help, and your self. Claim rest and private space without apology. None of this is stolen from your partner. A supporter with reserves is a better partner, and a supporter with nothing left is no use to anyone, least of all the person they are emptying themselves for.

There is one more chapter, and it is the most serious in the book. Everything so far has assumed a relationship that is difficult but fundamentally safe, in which the trauma strains the bond but does not endanger you. That is not every relationship. Sometimes what looks like a partner's trauma tips into coercion, threat, or violence, and support becomes something else entirely. The final chapter draws the line that every other chapter depends on: understanding why a person behaves as they do is never the same as accepting behavior that is unsafe, and love does not require you to live in danger.

Chapter 10: Love Does Not Require Unsafe Conditions

Elorien knew every reason. She could explain her partner Orlian's behavior better than anyone, because she had spent three years learning to. The checking of her phone was because his trust had been shattered by betrayal in childhood. The rage when she came home late was fear of abandonment. The way he decided who she could see, how she spent money, what she wore, was his need for control in a world that had once stripped all control from him. The night he grabbed her arm hard enough to leave marks, that was a flashback, he said, he had not known it was her. Elorien understood all of it. Understanding it was how she had stayed. And understanding it was, she finally saw, not the same as being safe, because no explanation had ever made the marks stop appearing.

This chapter is different from the others, and it may be the most important one in the book. Everything up to now has assumed a relationship that is hard but fundamentally safe, in which trauma strains the bond without endangering you. For some readers, that assumption holds, and this chapter will be a boundary line you are glad to know exists but do not need to cross. For others, it will name something you have been explaining away for a long time. Either way, the line has to be drawn clearly, because it is the line that makes every other chapter in this book true. Love does not require you to live in danger.

Understanding is not the same as accepting

The central skill of this whole book has been understanding, learning why your partner behaves as they do, so you can respond with compassion rather than blame. That skill has a shadow side, and this is the chapter where we face it. Understanding why a behavior happens is not the same as accepting it, and the two get fatally confused when the behavior is harmful. You can fully understand that your partner's control comes from their trauma, and still refuse to be controlled. You can grasp exactly why the rage erupts, and still decline to live inside it. The reason is never the same as permission.

This distinction matters because trauma is often used, sometimes by the partner and sometimes by the supporting partner's own compassion, as an explanation that quietly becomes an excuse. "He didn't mean it, it was a flashback." "She only does it because of what happened to her." These may even be true as explanations. They are never sufficient as permission, because your safety does not depend on whether the harm was intended or explicable. Harm is harm, and its cause, however sympathetic, does not change what it does to you. A person can be genuinely traumatized and genuinely unsafe to live with, and holding both of those truths at once is what keeps a compassionate partner from staying too long in a situation that is hurting them.

Safety Is the Floor. Understanding why harm happens is never the same as accepting it. Compassion for the cause does not obligate you to endure the effect, and no explanation, however true, requires you to live in danger.

Trauma symptoms and abuse are not the same thing

It is important to be careful and fair here, because this book has spent nine chapters insisting that people with trauma are not burdens or dangers, and that remains true. Most people with post-traumatic stress are not abusive. Their symptoms may make them withdrawn, irritable, anxious, or hard to reach, and those things are difficult to live alongside, but they are not the same as abuse, and it would be a serious error to read this chapter as suggesting that a trauma survivor is a threat. Vaelan's wife Aeris, from the first chapter, has real symptoms and has never once endangered him. That is the ordinary case.

Abuse is a different phenomenon, and it has a recognizable shape. Researchers describe a pattern called coercive control, in which one person systematically dominates another through isolation, intimidation, monitoring, control of money and movement, threats, and sometimes physical or sexual violence, all of which work together to strip away the other person's freedom and sense of self (Stark, 2007). The distinguishing feature is not the presence of trauma but the presence of control and fear. Trauma symptoms are something your partner struggles with. Coercive control is something done to you, systematically, in a way that makes you smaller and more afraid over time. The test is not whether your partner has a painful history. The test is whether you are being controlled and harmed, and whether you are afraid.

The questions that cut through

When compassion has been explaining harm for a long time, it can be genuinely hard to see your own situation clearly, because you have built an entire framework for interpreting every incident charitably. A few plain questions can cut through that framework, and they are worth asking yourself plainly, in private.

Are you afraid of your partner. Do you change your behavior, your words, your movements, to avoid their anger. Has physical force been used against you, even once, even with an explanation attached. Are you isolated from friends and family, cut off from money, monitored, or controlled in where you go and what you do. Do you feel smaller, more frightened, and less yourself than you did before this relationship. Have threats been made, against you, against themselves, or against others, to keep you in line. These questions are not about whether your partner is a good or bad person, and they are not about their trauma. They are about your safety and your freedom, which are the only things this chapter is measuring. If the real answers point toward fear and control, that is information you cannot afford to explain away, no matter how well you understand the cause.

Threats to self are not a leash

There is one form of coercion that traps compassionate partners more than any other, and it must be named directly. Sometimes a partner uses the threat of self-harm to prevent you from leaving, from setting boundaries, or from having a life of your own. "If you go, I don't know what I'll do." "If you leave me, I won't survive it." This is one of the most agonizing situations a supporting partner can face, because the fear is real and the love is real and the stakes feel unbearable.

Here is what has to be said clearly. You are not responsible for another adult's survival, and you cannot keep a person alive by surrendering your own life to them, and staying in response to such threats does not actually keep anyone safe. If your partner is genuinely at risk of harming themselves, that is a medical emergency that requires professionals, crisis services, and their treatment team, not a reason for you to abandon your boundaries or remain in a situation that is destroying you. The compassionate and the responsible response to a threat of self-harm is the same: take it seriously, involve professionals and emergency services as appropriate, and refuse to let it become a leash. You can care deeply about your partner's life and still refuse to be held hostage by the threat of its ending. If you or your partner are in crisis, contact local emergency services or a crisis line right away; in the United States you can call or text 988 for the Suicide and Crisis Lifeline.

If you need to leave, leave carefully

If you recognize your own relationship in the pattern of coercive control, the most important thing to know is that leaving an abusive relationship is a specialized situation that you should not try to plan alone. The period around leaving can be the most dangerous time, and safety planning is genuinely a skill that trained advocates have and you likely do not. This is not a moment for a self-help book to give you a procedure. It is a moment to get expert help.

What a book can do is point you toward that help and encourage you to reach for it. Domestic violence hotlines and advocates can help you assess your situation, think through safety, and plan next steps in a way that is tailored to your specific circumstances, and there is good evidence that this kind of support helps people move toward safety (Stark, 2007). In the United States, the National Domestic Violence Hotline can be reached at 800-799-7233, and it offers confidential support; services and their exact terms vary, so it is worth confirming what is available in your area. If you are in immediate danger, contact emergency services. None of this requires you to have decided anything yet. You can talk to an advocate simply to understand your options, before you know what you want to do. Reaching out for that conversation is not a betrayal of your partner or your love. It is the point at which self-preservation has to come first.

A note on this chapter's exercise. The other chapters ended with things to try this week. This one ends differently, on purpose. If any part of this chapter has described your life, the action is not a journaling prompt. It is to talk, confidentially, to a professional who understands abuse, a domestic violence advocate, a therapist, or a crisis line, about what you are living with. That is the step. Please take it, when it is safe to do so, and take it before you try to decide anything on your own.

What happened to Elorien

Elorien did not leave the first time she saw the pattern clearly, or the second. Recognizing coercive control and acting on it are two different things, separated, often, by a long and frightening distance, and it does no one any good to pretend leaving is simple. What changed for Elorien was a single confidential phone call to a domestic violence advocate, made from a parking lot on her lunch break, in which she described her life out loud to someone trained to hear it and was told, gently and without pressure, that what she was describing was abuse and that help existed. She did not decide anything on that call. She just stopped being alone with it.

Months later, with the advocate's help and a careful plan she did not make by herself, Elorien left, safely. It was the hardest thing she had ever done, and she grieved Orlian even as she went, because understanding him had never stopped, and the love had been real. Both things were true. She loved him, and she could not be safe with him, and in the end safety had to be the floor. That is not a failure of compassion. It is compassion that finally included herself.

When you are not sure it counts

Not everyone who reads this chapter will recognize a clear-cut case. Many supporting partners live in a gray zone, where some things are frightening and some are not, where the harm is real but intermittent, where they genuinely cannot tell whether what they are experiencing is trauma symptoms they should meet with compassion or abuse they should not tolerate. If that is you, the uncertainty itself is worth taking seriously rather than using as a reason to wait indefinitely.

Here is a gentle principle for the gray zone. You do not have to be certain that your situation is abuse in order to talk to someone about it. You do not have to have proof, or a name for it, or a decision already made. Confidential support from a professional who understands these dynamics exists precisely for people who are not sure, and one of its purposes is to help you see your own situation more clearly than you can from inside it. If you find yourself minimizing, explaining away, or hoping you are overreacting, those very reflexes are worth mentioning to someone trained to hear them, because they are common in exactly the situations that turn out to matter most.

Trust your fear more than your explanations. Supporting partners in this book have been praised, chapter after chapter, for their capacity to understand, and that capacity is a strength almost everywhere. In the presence of possible danger, it can become a liability, because a mind skilled at understanding can explain away almost anything, including its own alarm. If some part of you is afraid, and keeps being afraid, and keeps talking itself out of the fear, that pattern is information. You are allowed to take your own fear seriously even when you can construct a compassionate explanation for what causes it. The explanation and the danger can both be real, and your safety is measured by the danger, not by the sympathy of its cause.

None of this is a push toward any particular decision. It is a push toward one conversation, held with someone who understands abuse, in which you are allowed to be uncertain and are helped to see clearly. Whatever you decide afterward is yours. But please do not let the fact that your situation is ambiguous, or that you love your partner, or that you understand exactly why they are the way they are, keep you from the one conversation that could tell you whether the floor beneath your relationship is safety or something else.

The through-line, and the end of the road

Understanding why a person harms you is never the same as accepting the harm, and no explanation, however true, obligates you to live in danger. Trauma symptoms are not the same as abuse; the difference is control and fear. If you are afraid, controlled, or harmed, those are facts your compassion cannot be allowed to explain away, and if you are being held by the threat of a partner's self-harm, that is a matter for professionals rather than a reason to surrender your life. Leaving an abusive relationship is a specialized task that trained advocates should help you plan. And love, real love, does not require unsafe conditions, because a person who is being destroyed cannot love well, and was never meant to.

This is where the road this book has walked comes to its end. You began by seeing a job you never applied for. You learned to pull apart the roles you were never meant to hold all at once, to step out of the rescue loop, to help without taking over, to set boundaries built on your own land, to survive the guilt that follows them, to open the door to treatment without becoming the treatment, to keep love running in both directions, and to build the support that a supporter needs. And you learned, finally, where the whole thing rests: on safety, on the plain refusal to call danger love. Take what serves you and leave the rest. Somewhere in all of this is the version of you who loves this person and still has a self. That version was never gone. You have been walking back toward them the whole way.

A Final Word

If you have read this far, you have done a quieter kind of hard work than the world usually notices. Not the loud work of a crisis, but the slow work of looking clearly at a role you never chose and deciding, piece by piece, to hold it differently. That deserves to be named, because no one else is likely to name it for you.

I want to be candid with you at the end, the way I have tried to be throughout. Nothing in this book resolves in a straight line. You will set a boundary and then abandon it, catch yourself in the rescue loop after you swore you were done, slide back into the clinician's chair on a hard night, and lose an evening to guilt you know is not a verdict. That is not failure. That is what change looks like when it is real. Progress in this territory is not a clean climb. It is a long series of noticing, slipping, and returning, and the returning is the whole skill. You do not have to do any of it perfectly. You only have to keep coming back to it.

If there is one thing I hope you carry out of these pages, it is the plainest idea in the book: some things are yours, some are your partner's, and some belong to the two of you together, and most of your exhaustion has come from carrying items that were never in your column. You can keep loving your partner and set some of that weight down. The love does not require the weight. It never did.

This is a handoff, not a finish line. Your relationship will keep changing, and so will you, and there will be seasons when you need to reread a chapter or reach for help you have not needed before. That is not backsliding. That is a life. Take what has served you here, leave what has not, and go on being the person who loves this person and still, at last, has a self.

Recommended Next Steps

This book is a beginning, not a complete plan, and it was never meant to be your only resource. The most useful next step for many readers is professional support of your own. A therapist or counselor who understands trauma and relationships can help you apply these ideas to the specific texture of your life, sort out your guilt and your boundaries, and put down the load for an hour with someone trained to hold it. If you have never considered therapy for yourself, on the grounds that your partner is the one with the diagnosis, let this be the nudge. Your wellbeing is worth its own care.

Consider a support group for partners and family members of trauma survivors. There is a particular relief in sitting among people who understand the specific loneliness of loving someone with a trauma history, and who will not expect you to be the strong one. Many such groups are low cost or free, offered through community organizations, veterans' services, and mental health centers. Finding one that fits your situation is a concrete step worth taking this month.

If your partner is open to it, couple-based approaches led by a qualified professional can help the two of you work on how trauma is affecting the relationship, together, rather than leaving the whole task to you. This is different from you delivering treatment at home. It is a trained professional guiding a shared process, and for some couples it changes what feels possible.

For further reading, look for books grounded in the research rather than in slogans, and prefer authors with genuine clinical or scholarly credentials. The References section that follows lists the sources this book drew on, and several of them, particularly the accessible books, are worth seeking out if you want to go deeper into a specific area.

Finally, if anything in the last chapter described your life, please make the professional conversation about safety your first next step, ahead of everything else on this page. A domestic violence advocate or crisis line can help you understand your situation and your options confidentially, before you decide anything. In the United States, the National Domestic Violence Hotline can be reached at 800-799-7233, and the Suicide and Crisis Lifeline at 988. Confirm current local resources for your area, and if you are in immediate danger, contact emergency services. Your safety comes before every other step in this book.

References

Allen, E. S., Renshaw, K. D., Fredman, S. J., Le, Y., Rhoades, G. K., Markman, H. J., & Litz, B. T. (2021). Associations between service members' posttraumatic stress disorder symptoms and partner accommodation over time. *Journal of Traumatic Stress, 34*(3), 596-606. https://doi.org/10.1002/jts.22645

Deci, E. L., & Ryan, R. M. (2000). The "what" and "why" of goal pursuits: Human needs and the self-determination of behavior. *Psychological Inquiry, 11*(4), 227-268. https://doi.org/10.1207/S15327965PLI1104_01

Fredman, S. J., Le, Y., Renshaw, K. D., & Allen, E. S. (2022). Longitudinal associations among service members' PTSD symptoms, partner accommodation, and partner distress. *Behavior Therapy, 53*(6), 1161-1174. https://doi.org/10.1016/j.beth.2022.05.005

Fredman, S. J., Vorstenbosch, V., Wagner, A. C., Macdonald, A., & Monson, C. M. (2014). Partner accommodation in posttraumatic stress disorder: Initial testing of the Significant Others' Responses to Trauma Scale (SORTS). *Journal of Anxiety Disorders, 28*(4), 372-381. https://doi.org/10.1016/j.janxdis.2014.04.001

Herman, J. L. (2015). *Trauma and recovery: The aftermath of violence, from domestic abuse to political terror* (Rev. ed.). Basic Books. (Original work published 1992)

Hochschild, A. R. (1983). *The managed heart: Commercialization of human feeling.* University of California Press.

Miller, W. R., & Rollnick, S. (2013). *Motivational interviewing: Helping people change* (3rd ed.). Guilford Press.

Monson, C. M., & Fredman, S. J. (2012). *Cognitive-behavioral conjoint therapy for PTSD: Harnessing the healing power of relationships.* Guilford Press.

Neff, K. D. (2003). The development and validation of a scale to measure self-compassion. *Self and Identity, 2*(3), 223-250. https://doi.org/10.1080/15298860309027

Neff, K. D. (2023). Self-compassion: Theory, method, research, and intervention. *Annual Review of Psychology, 74*, 193-218. https://doi.org/10.1146/annurev-psych-032420-031047

Nelson Goff, B. S., & Smith, D. B. (2005). Systemic traumatic stress: The Couple Adaptation to Traumatic Stress Model. *Journal of Marital and Family Therapy, 31*(2), 145-157. https://doi.org/10.1111/j.1752-0606.2005.tb01552.x

Pukay-Martin, N. D., Torbit, L., Landy, M. S. H., Wanklyn, S. G., Shnaider, P., Lane, J. E. M., & Monson, C. M. (2015). An uncontrolled trial of a present-focused cognitive-behavioral conjoint therapy for posttraumatic stress disorder. *Journal of Clinical Psychology, 71*(4), 302-312. https://doi.org/10.1002/jclp.22166

Renshaw, K. D., Allen, E. S., Fredman, S. J., Giff, S. T., & Kern, C. (2020). Partners' motivations for accommodating posttraumatic stress disorder symptoms in service members: The Reasons for Accommodation of PTSD Scale. *Journal of Anxiety Disorders, 71*, 102199. https://doi.org/10.1016/j.janxdis.2020.102199

Stark, E. (2007). *Coercive control: How men entrap women in personal life.* Oxford University Press.

World Health Organization. (2019). *International classification of diseases for mortality and morbidity statistics* (11th ed.). https://icd.who.int/

www.ingramcontent.com/pod-product-compliance
Lightning Source LLC
LaVergne TN
LVHW050827061126
851857LV00012B/1016
* 9 7 9 8 9 0 6 7 8 1 7 2 7 *